Heamatologist - blood specialist

Endocrinology - glands
thyroid & hypothyroid

pg 113 crippling disease

Narcolepsy - sleep disorder pg 130

10-15-79

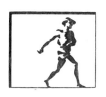

BOOKS BY LAWRENCE GALTON

The Complete Medical, Fitness & Health Guide for Men
The Complete Medical Guide, *with Benjamin F. Miller, M.D.*
The Family Book of Preventive Medicine, *with Benjamin F. Miller, M.D.*
Freedom from Heart Attacks, *with Benjamin F. Miller, M.D.*
Freedom from Backaches, *with Lawrence W. Friedmann, M.D.*
Your Inner Conflicts, *with W. Hugh Missildine, M.D.*
How Long Will I Live?
The Laboratory of the Body
Medical Advances
Save Your Stomach
The Truth About Fiber in Your Food
Don't Give Up on an Aging Parent
The Silent Disease: Hypertension
The Disguised Disease: Anemia
Hypothyroidism: The Unsuspected Illness, *with Broda O. Barnes, M.D.*
Adult Physical Fitness Manual, The President's Council on Physical Fitness

YOU MAY NOT NEED A PSYCHIATRIST

How Your Body May Control Your Mind

LAWRENCE GALTON

SIMON AND SCHUSTER NEW YORK

Published by Simon and Schuster
A Division of Gulf & Western Corporation
Simon & Schuster Building
Rockefeller Center
1230 Avenue of the Americas
New York, New York 10020
Designed by Edith Fowler
Manufactured in the United States of America

1 2 3 4 5 6 7 8 9 10

Library of Congress Cataloging in Publication Data

Galton, Lawrence.
You may not need a psychiatrist

Includes bibliographical references and index.
1. Psychology, Physiological. 2. Depression, Mental. 3. Stress (Psychology) 4. Anxiety. I. Title.
QP360.G34 616.8'5 79-324

ISBN 0-671-24240-7

Acknowledgments

To the many investigators noted in the Selected References whose work has helped to focus my attention, and hopefully that of more and more in the medical profession, on the subject of this book. And especially to the following, whose special, helpful courtesies contributed much to making this book possible:

M. Brent Campbell, M.D., Vista Hill Hospital, San Diego
Norman Geschwind, M.D., Harvard Medical School and Beth Israel Hospital, Boston
John F. Greden, M.D., University of Michigan
Richard C. W. Hall, M.D., University of Texas
Luis V. M. Huapaya, M.D., McGill University
David J. Kupfer, M.D., University of Pittsburgh
John LaWall, M.D., University of Arizona
Brendan A. Maher, Ph. D., Harvard University
Marshall Mandell, M.D., New York Medical College
W. H. Philpott, M.D., Ecology House Clinic & Laboratory, Oklahoma City
Arthur C. Walsh, M.D., University of Pittsburgh

Contents

1. Overview: But Is It—So Much—in the Mind? A Matter of Nerves? Psychogenic? Psychosomatic?

It has been fashionable now for years—in medical and lay circles—to think of much illness as psychogenic.

The idea has become so firmly entrenched that not just cocktail party/backyard chatter but serious statements in the medical literature, repeatedly made, would have it that one-half, two-thirds, even 70 percent of all patients consulting physicians have nothing physically wrong but are victims of "functional" disorders, of "in the mind" disturbances that upset mind or body or both.

Have we—and many of our physicians—become too enamored of the concept? Too dangerously ready to accept its glib application? At high economic cost? At the expense of much useless treatment? And of much needless suffering?

- A 33-year-old attorney suffers from unrelenting fatigue, shops many physicians, is consigned to the psychoneurotic category, tries psychotherapy, gets no help. Finally: a long-neglected check for hypothyroidism. Thyroid therapy ends the fatigue.

- A 25-year-old woman seems to be a victim of anxiety neurosis because of episodes of great, nameless apprehension, often accompanied by sweats, palpitation, vomiting, diarrhea. Her real problem: paroxysmal tachycardia, a heart rhythm disturbance. Quinidine treatment restores normal rhythm; the "anxiety neurosis" disappears.

- A gray-haired housewife seems a classic case of severe mental depression—unresponsive, apathetic, face sagging expressionlessly—until neurologists, taking a closer look, find a brain tumor, remove it, and she recovers completely.

- A middle-aged man is found sitting in his room barking like a dog, apparently schizophrenic. He is quickly committed to a psychiatric unit. But further examination reveals Parkinsonism, which can produce a barklike respiratory tic. He responds to treatment for the physical disease, goes home well.

- A 24-year-old man is brought grunting, rolling, rocking, sucking, blowing, and grinning to an emergency room. It's the thirtieth time in five years; the staff knows exactly what to do. Three hours after a stiff dose of a powerful tranquilizer the man rubs his eyes as if just awakening, asks calmly for a cigarette. Mentally deranged? No. Finally, five years late, a complete study shows psychomotor epilepsy with "complex partial seizures." Anticonvulsant medicine now keeps him well.

- After four hospitalizations for suicidal attempts between ages 13 and 16, an adolescent girl has to be kept in a sanitarium for three years, unresponsive to shock or other treatment. Finally, allergy tests are carried out and severe hypersensitivities are discovered. Among them: saccharin, which makes her dizzy and anxious; chlorine-treated water, which makes her depressed; lamb, which causes sweating, confusion, crying. With the allergens avoided, she regains equilibrium, has no symptom recurrences, enters college.

- A New York City judge, after a first sudden episode of confusion, disorientation, and severe headache, deteriorates progressively for two years, becoming anxious, depressed, and paranoic. Forty-eight hours after he is found to have occult hydrocephalus (water on the brain) and the condition is surgically corrected, he is alert, cheerful, oriented.

This is a small sampling of cases to be found in this book.

Does psychosomatic illness exist? Of course. Emotional disorders can, indeed, cause behavioral disturbances and physical illness.

But the reverse is true and too often goes unsuspected: overlooked physical illness—not obvious, not instantly detectable—can be responsible for emotional and behavioral disturbances and, moreover, for many seemingly psychogenic physical symptoms.

In a recent study by University of Texas and University of Minnesota Medical School investigators, the masking of underlying physical disorders by psychiatric symptoms was found to be a common problem, commonly unappreciated, not only by patients but by physicians.

Recently, too, Boston's Beth Israel Hospital, a teaching institution affiliated with Harvard Medical School, thought it necessary to set up a special Behavioral Neurology Unit. A major purpose: to spot and treat patients with many conditions often misdiagnosed as psychological in origin.

"There are probably more misdiagnoses in this field than in any other," observes Dr. Norman Geschwind, director of the Unit and professor of neurology at Harvard.

At a recent annual meeting and scientific assembly, the American Society of Contemporary Medicine and Surgery organized a special course for its twelve thousand physician members on "Neuropsychiatric Manifestations of Systemic Disease."

If some current estimates are correct, as many as 120,000—40 percent—of the 300,000 hospitalized mental patients in the United States may be victims not of emotional illnesses but of physical disorders that affect behavior.

Nobody knows how many hundreds of thousands, or possibly millions, of the nonhospitalized with a diversity of so-called "psychogenic," "psychosomatic," or "it's just your nerves" problems are victims of undetected and remediable physical disorders.

They include many suffering from excessive fatigue, weakness, anxiety states, depressed feelings, irritability, concentration difficulties, memory disturbances, personality changes, delusional thinking, and many with strange fevers, head pains, joint pains, gastrointestinal and still other physical symptoms.

What, hopefully, can a book such as this do for them?

Possibly it can encourage many who haven't ever sought help, including those who have believed that the reason for their problems had to lie deep in the subconscious, with a solution possible only through extended psychiatric treatment they could not afford or preferred not to face.

Possibly it can alert them, and others who have sought help unsuccessfully in the past, so that when they seek help now they can be aware of and can suggest physical possibilities, even perhaps specific ones, to physicians—possibilities that might otherwise escape consideration.

Possibly it can help some not only to figure out what may be wrong but even in some cases to set it right—those, for example, whose seemingly emotionally based difficulties may stem from allergies, nutritional problems, or medications either self- or physician-prescribed.

2. *Psychosomatic, Yes . . . but Somatopsychic Too*

The word "psychosomatic" is only about half a century old. It first appeared in the German medical literature in the early 1920's. A decade later, Dr. Helen Flanders Dunbar of Columbia University College of Physicians and Surgeons used it in her book *Emotions and Bodily Changes,* which was to become a classic. It wasn't long before "psychosomatic" came into common use.

It means, of course, that the mind can influence the body, that emotional problems can cause physical disturbances. And although the word is new, the concept is not.

More than four thousand years ago, Chinese physicians observed that physical illness could follow frustration. Half a millennium before the birth of Christ, Hippocrates, father of medicine, cautioned that physicians, if they were to bring about cures, would need to have a knowledge "of the whole of things," of mind as well as body. Ancient Roman physicians used a form of psychotherapy as an aid in relieving bodily suffering.

Throughout the Middle Ages, emotional influences in disease were recognized. But then, late in the nineteenth century, as specific microorganisms were found to be agents of many diseases and the germ theory of illness flourished, emotional factors were overshadowed.

More recently, however, the pendulum has swung the other way.

There have been studies in recent years which have suggested that while germs undoubtedly cause such afflictions as the common cold and skin, gastrointestinal, and many other infections, an individual's susceptibility to germ activity may rise or fall depending upon his or her state of mind.

Many studies have suggested possible links between state of mind and many other kinds of diseases, even including cancer.

One investigation, for example, considered the case of a hardworking, phlegmatic Midwestern housewife who for twenty years had cared for a mentally retarded daughter. She took it stoically when the daughter died. She took it stoically, too, when, a few months later, another daughter married against her parents' wishes and cut herself off from the family. A few months after that, the woman, never sick in her life, collapsed and was dead of cancer within a month.

She had suffered two great losses and had refused to discuss them and discuss her feelings. Was her own death from cancer coincidental? Not to investigators who had noted similar coincidences in the lives of hundreds of cancer patients in studies suggesting that the way a person handles emotional problems somehow may set the stage for cancer development.

In a study in Scotland, when two hundred lung cancer patients were compared with two hundred other persons without cancer, the cancer patients were found to be less emotionally reactive and without outlets for emotional release.

Dr. Sydney G. Margolin of the University of Colorado has observed that the Sioux Indians, whom he describes as having few emotional inhibitions, are almost completely free of cancer. And several cross-cultural investigations have suggested that in countries where cancer death rates are high, emotional inhibition is common.

Emotional repression and emotional "give up"

According to Dr. C. B. Bahnson, professor of psychiatry at Jefferson Medical College, Philadelphia, emotions themselves do not cause cancer but may set the stage for growth of malignant cells. "When a loss occurs, rather than going through a typical cathartic mourning process," he notes, "these [cancer-prone] persons tend to deny the loss, adopt a Pollyanna attitude that says everything is fine, and keep on with their activities as if nothing had happened. Instead of their emotions being expressed in behavior, they go through the central nervous system which in turn affects the body hormones and immune responses in such a way as to permit the development of cancer."

In the course of a large research program into emotion-body relationships at the University of Rochester, Drs. George L. Engel and Arthur Schmale have found that many patients hospitalized for a physical illness have had a psychological disturbance shortly before they got sick.

Most commonly, the patients had experienced an attitude of helplessness, of giving up. As some expressed it, "It was just too much; I couldn't take any more." The helpless feeling usually followed loss or threat of loss of someone or something close to the patient—a spouse, parent, child, home, job, or planned career.

The suggestion from thousands of patient interviews in the Rochester study is that if a person responds to some significant event in his life with a feeling of hopelessness, helplessness, or giving up, he may somehow trigger a biological change that may promote the development of an already-existing disease potential.

In one Rochester investigation, Dr. Schmale and a colleague, Dr. Howard P. Iker, found that they could predict with 75 percent accuracy the presence of cancer based on psychiatric interviews with fifty-one women appearing at the Medical Center for cervical biopsies. All had had Pap smear tests indicating possible malignancy. The two physicians predicted that eighteen who had responded to some recent situation in their lives with hopeless feelings would turn out to actually have cancer. Of the eighteen, eleven in fact did have it. Of thirty-three predicted to be free of cancer, twenty-five did not have it.

To explain such findings, Dr. Schmale suggests: "Man is constantly interacting with his many environments, and at many levels of organization—from the subcellular and biochemical to the most external or peripheral, that of family, work, and now even his universe. We postulate that when a person gives up psychologically he is disrupting the continuity of his relatedness to himself and his many environments or levels of organization. In making such a break, or with this loss of continuity, he may become more vulnerable to the pathogenic influences in his external environment and/or he may become more cut off from his external environments and more predisposed to internal derangements. Thus, disease is more apt to appear at such time of disruptions and increased vulnerability."

And Dr. Engel notes that it is not so much the magnitude of an event as how a person reacts to it that determines whether he gives up. A seemingly minor event, such as loss of a pet, may to some people be the last straw, whereas others would not give up even after loss of family, home, or job.

Personality types and illnesses

Some investigators, notably Dr. Franz Alexander and his colleagues at the Chicago Institute for Psychoanalysis, have suggested that specific personality types may be prone to specific diseases.

For example, they see the typical rheumatoid arthritis sufferer as one who has difficulty handling hostile and aggressive feelings and who tries to curb them, using great self-control but also exercising a kind of benevolent tyranny over others. The arthritis may be triggered when there is a loss of a person who has been dominated.

Asthmatics seem to be in another category. At least, in

many cases, the Chicago research suggests, as children they inhibited their crying for fear of being rejected, particularly by their mothers. And they grew up with a frustrated desire to cry, which may be manifested by a frustration of breathing—asthma.

The person with high blood pressure, according to the Chicago findings, often is one who swallows his hostilities, has difficulty asserting himself, tends to be overly responsible, works hard and doggedly, feels increasing resentment, and lives in a state of tension.

It must be said that the Chicago findings are no longer as widely accepted as they once were. To many now, they seem untenable because of newer insights into disease. For example, the Alexander group considered that the curbed hostility of the rheumatoid arthritis patient produced increased tension in the joint muscles, leading to arthritic lesions, but it is now known that the muscle tension actually arises because of the painful joint inflammation.

On the other hand, another disease, coronary artery disease, not included by the Alexander group among personality-influenced, has in recent years been the subject of considerable interest. A series of studies has suggested that people with a particular personality constellation are more prone to develop coronary artery disease, which is a forerunner of heart attacks. The personality constellation, called the Type A, includes such features as urgency about and excessive consciousness of deadlines, a driven quality of speech, and a tendency to be impatient.

The Type A individual is so aggressive that even when he plays games with his children, he plays to win. He loves to compete with fellow workers, would much rather have the respect of associates than their affection.

One of the most distinguishing features of the A person is inability to be satisfied with achievements accompanied by a huge need to try to get more and more done in a given period.

Extreme A people can go to ridiculous lengths to get more things done. Says Dr. Meyer Friedman, the San Francisco cardiologist who pioneered the studies of A personalities: "Some subjects like to evacuate their bowels, read the financial section of the newspaper, and shave with an electric razor, all at the same time. One subject admitted that he had already purchased ten different electric razors in his efforts to find one that would shave faster than all others, and another subject liked to use two electric razors at the same time so he could cut his shaving time in half."

In distinction, the B person may be just as serious but is much more easygoing, able to enjoy leisure, with no feelings of being driven by time. He can be ambitious but in a quiet, more reasonable way. He is easier to get along with, harder to anger.

In one of many studies by Dr. Friedman, indicating the propensity of A people to develop heart trouble, 3,500 men, aged 39 to 59, all with no indication of heart disease, were interviewed and classified as Type A or B. Four years later, fifty-two had developed a first heart attack and eighteen a first attack of anginal chest pain indicating coronary heart disease. The incidence of the disease was three times greater among the Type A than among the Type B men. Some years later, when 257 of the men had developed coronary heart disease, 70 percent of the victims were Type A.

When a similar study was carried out with women—most but not all the A women worked in industry or in professional jobs; most but not all the B were housewives—the A women developed more coronary heart disease (19 percent) than the B women (4 percent).

Stress effects

To no small extent, Type A people make their own emotional stress. Whether or not self-made, emotional stress has been shown in many studies to have physical effects.

Stress reactions are the body's set of involuntary responses to the demands of living, to dangers or even seeming dangers that may arise in living. Early man needed these instantaneous, unthinking reactions to survive. They mustered his physical resources to meet threats. When he suddenly encountered a wild beast, he had to fight or flee, and, for either, needed an extra surge of strength. Immediately, his body accommodated. Reacting to the stress, it caused extra amounts of hormones from his adrenal glands to pour into his blood; raised his pulse rate, breathing, and blood pressure; mobilized energy from sugar and stored fats and dispatched it to his muscles and brain; and turned off any digestive processes going on so they would not use up energy.

Although modern man rarely today is presented with situations calling for fighting or fleeing, he has the same old set of stress reactions. And they can be triggered by situations that make him fearful, anxious, frustrated. If he sees something as a threat to his job, if he reacts with frustration to a traffic tie-up, if he becomes provoked by spouse or child, out pour the adrenal hormones and the stress reactions are activated. But there is no physical outlet for the extra energy; it is bottled up.

And if he develops chronic patterns of stress, he may pay a physical price. Under more or less continuous stress, some vital body parts may be disrupted, leading to illness.

The whole concept of harmful stress was developed by Dr. Hans Selye, director of the Institute of Experimental Medicine and Surgery at the University of Montreal, who exposed laboratory animals to varied stressful situations: extremes of temperature, loud noises, frustrating situations such as being tied spread-eagled to a board.

No matter what the stress inducer, if it had to be endured for prolonged periods, it wreaked havoc. Upon autopsy, the animals were found to have peptic ulcers, enlarged adrenal glands, disturbances in other body organs.

According to Dr. Selye, there are three stages of stress. In the first, an alarm stage, the body reacts to a stress that can be a physical one or an emotional one, such as nervous tension. Then comes a second stage in which hormones pour out and energy is maintained at a high level to deal with the stressful situation. But this is supercharged living. If it is maintained over a long period, the third stage—exhaustion—sets in and one or more body organs may be impaired.

Since Selye first developed the concept in 1950, evidence has accumulated on how stress, notably emotional stress, may play a significant role in coronary heart disease in particular.

One way is through elevation of blood cholesterol levels, considered to be an important coronary heart disease risk factor. Studies have shown that students preparing for final examinations and income tax accountants under heavy pressure just before tax deadline time have higher cholesterol levels during such periods than at other times. Studies with Air Force personnel have shown higher cholesterol levels during stressful than in nonstress periods. In Navy underwater demolition trainees tested repeatedly during training, cholesterol levels were found to rise whenever they were angry, depressed, or fearful.

High blood pressure, excess weight, lack of exercise, cigarette smoking, and diabetes also rank high among risk factors for coronary heart disease. Consider, then, suggests cardiologist-researcher Dr. Henry I. Russek, that "it is well recognized that emotional tension may result in compulsive eating, drinking and smoking, in many persons as compensation for anxiety. Moreover, it does frequently contribute to the failure to achieve daily exercise by promoting fatigue, creating a sense of time urgency, and decreasing motivation. Nervous strain of occupational, cultural, social, or domestic origin is known to elevate blood pressure, to increase the tendency to obesity, to contribute to excessive smoking and lack of exercise, to participate in hypercholesterolemia [high cholesterol levels], and aggravate diabetes through psychic influences. . . . Even such indirect effects of emotional stress, barring all others, must elevate this factor to a position of considerable significance in coronary heart disease."

Nothing in this book is meant to gainsay the possible importance of emotion in disease—in many kinds of disease. Nor is there any intention to downplay the importance of finding constructive ways of handling potentially threatening emotional influences and behavior.

It is certainly no simple matter to change one's personality and behavior pattern. But it would seem that anything at all an A person can do to relax even just a little, to stop constantly cramming more and more activities into his or her life, could be helpful.

Stress is unavoidable—an integral part of living. Extreme A people complicate matters by adding extra stress to their lives. But everybody faces stress and it is not necessarily bad. It only becomes so when it is protracted and unrelieved.

A few fortunate people have the ability to take even excessively stressful situations in stride, avoiding excessive reactions to them. Anyone without that ability may find it wise if faced, for example, with a continuously frustrating job, to quit and get another, however much of a wrench that may mean. Better the wrench than facing a possibility of disabling or deadly illness.

There are many possible maneuvers that may help ameliorate stress. Dr. Selye recalls that "once when I was about six years old I was crying, miserable. What brought it on, I do not remember. My grandmother was sympathetic—and wise. 'Go to the mirror,' she said, 'and smile with your face. Soon you will be smiling all over.' Curiously enough, it worked—and was less stressful than pounding my head against a wall."

Distraction can be good medicine—reading, listening to music, seeing a movie, watching a television program, in fact almost anything that takes one's mind off a stressful problem, even temporarily.

For years, wise physicians have known that exercise can do much to release tensions and distract from and even reduce turmoil. Dr. Paul Dudley White, the famed cardiologist, often remarked: "To get physically tired is the best antidote for nervous tension. In my own case, nervous tension and strain can be counteracted, even prevented, by regular exercise."

But Now—To the Somatopsychic

If emotional difficulties and disturbances can be involved, clearly enough and even commonly, in physical disorders, there is a need to recognize how commonly physical disturbances, apparent or not, may underlie emotional and behavioral disturbances.

"Somatopsychic" is no new coined word. You can find it in medical dictionaries, defined as "relating to the mind-body relationship; the study of the effects of the body upon the mind."

Yet, while psychosomatic has become a household word, somatopsychic is, to most people, strange.

It should be no surprise that, given mind-body unity, if mind may affect body, so may body affect mind.

And this, of course, is within the common experience of anyone who has ever had a bad cold and noted not only coughing, sneezing, and runny nose but such mental effects as irritability and gloominess as well.

It has been known for a long time—even if much more is known today—that psychiatric symptoms can develop when any condition disrupts the brain or alters its delicate functioning and that body disturbances can do this.

Before the days of penicillin, neurosyphilis was a major cause of mental hospitalization. As the disease progressed, it led to personality changes, irresponsible behavior, slovenly habits, memory defects, inability to concentrate. When far advanced, it could lead to mania.

Once, pellagra, a simple dietary deficiency of niacin, a B vitamin, led to bizarre behavioral symptoms. Among the first cases recognized in the United States were many in mental institutions—delirious, hallucinating, psychotic.

Once, too, brucellosis, an infectious disease transmitted by microorganisms in raw milk, was responsible for many cases of irritability, emotional instability, and mental depression.

Behavior disorders on an organic basis have also been known to stem from other causes. For example, when the hormones ACTH and cortisone were introduced in the early 1950's and used for arthritis and many other conditions, it quickly became apparent that many patients receiving high doses developed a variety of psychoses, complications less common today because of better control of dosage.

It is common knowledge, too, that many drugs such as alcohol, LSD, and the amphetamines may produce psychotic reactions.

It is, in fact, now known that a very wide variety of insults to the body can, through the body, become insults to the brain. The insults can be physical injuries; they can be physical diseases; they can be therapies of one kind or another used to combat the diseases; they can be nutritional deficiencies or disturbances; and, they can even, among other things, be sleep disturbances.

Indeed, the number of recognized physical problems capable of producing emotional and behavioral disturbances, seemingly psychiatric symptoms that often are the first or only signs of the underlying physical problems, has been growing.

But it has also become clear that for some years now, and continuing to today, all too often the body provokers of such disturbances, the somatopsychic influences, are overlooked, and there is a tendency among some physicians as well as many patients to leap to the conclusion that "it's all in the mind."

The overlooked

As far back as 1936, one investigator studying one hundred patients who had been labeled neurotic found that twenty-four developed significant physical disease within eight months after the initial neurotic diagnosis. It was important, he suggested, to consider that psychiatric and behavioral symptoms often could come before the full-blown development of obvious physical illness.

A dozen years later, another investigator discovered that

44 percent of a series of patients who had been admitted to a psychiatric unit had physical illness.

In the 1960's came a whole series of studies pointing up the fact that psychiatric symptoms are not specific, not limited to psychiatric disease, and commonly occur in medical, or physical, illnesses.

In one of the studies which covered 209 consecutive psychiatric patients, a 50 percent rate of physical illness was uncovered. In spite of previous medical examination, 5 percent of the patients had medical disorders that were considered clearly "causal" of their psychiatric symptoms. Twenty-one percent had significant medical illness which was considered "concomitant" and "apparently contributing" to the development of the psychological symptoms. Eight percent developed a physical disorder which "apparently" resulted either from the psychological illness or its treatment. And of the remaining patients, 34 percent were found to have physical illnesses that needed attention.

In another study of psychiatric patients, 42 percent were found to have physical disease that had caused their psychiatric complaints.

In still another, when detailed physical examinations were carried out on 250 consecutive patients admitted to an inpatient psychiatric service, 12 percent were found to have physical problems responsible for their psychiatric symptoms and 80 percent of these problems had been entirely missed by their physicians.

And in still another, 67 of 200 consecutive psychiatric inpatients carefully checked were found to have medical illness, with 70 percent of the illnesses considered severe and 49 percent of them previously unknown to either patient or physician.

There have been case reports, too, warning against glib assumptions that what appears to be psychiatric necessarily is.

One in 1974 told of a patient who complained of double vision, difficulty in swallowing and speaking, breathing difficulty, and general weakness. The symptoms were considered to be psychosomatic by many physicians before the diagnosis of botulism, the potentially fatal food poisoning, was made.

A report in 1976 described three patients with behavioral disturbances that had led to them being considered psychotic, and they were treated as such, until symptoms of viral encephalitis followed and it became evident that they were physically, not mentally, ill.

In a more recent study, by Drs. Richard C. W. Hall of the University of Texas Medical School and Michael K. Popkin of the University of Minnesota Medical School, 658 consecutive mental health outpatients were investigated and 9.1 percent were found to have a medical condition definitely or probably responsible for their psychiatric symptoms.

In these medically rather than emotionally ill patients, depression, anxiety, sleep disturbances, appetite disorders, diminished concentration, impaired recent memory, speech difficulty or a recent change of speech pattern, hallucinations (auditory or visual or both), and recent personality change were among the most characteristic psychiatric findings.

And in these patients, among the most frequent causes of the psychiatric symptoms were heart and blood vessel disease, endocrine gland disorders, infection, lung disease, gastrointestinal disease, blood problems, central nervous system disease, and cancer.

What the investigators considered especially noteworthy was that 28 percent of these patients had been diagnosed as psychotic. "These diagnoses carry with them the implication of long-term drug treatment, potential hospitalization, and possible changes in the patient's legal status. The majority of the patients diagnosed as being functionally psychotic cleared rapidly with appropriate medical treatment and remained healthy. Misdiagnosis and the application of psychiatric labels to medically ill patients reduces their chances for improvement and may result in a worsening of their physical health. Adequate medical investigation on the other hand is reassuring to both the patient and to his physician."

3. *Is It Really Mental Depression?*

He was a professional man in his late thirties who had experienced disturbing symptoms: chest pains that worried him that he might have heart disease; frequent headaches, seemingly out of the blue, unresponsive to usual remedies; loss of appetite; and difficulty in sleeping.

When he sought medical help, a thorough physical examination produced no clues. Nor did laboratory tests. The physician, however, was able to establish that the symptoms were not new; there had been several episodes, each a little more intensive and prolonged than the preceding one, and always accompanied by feelings of discouragement and despondency.

The diagnosis: depression.

The young housewife complained of almost overwhelming fatigue and almost constant abdominal distress. In her case, too, physical examination and testing failed to detect any organic disorder. Noting that she seemed withdrawn, passive, lethargic, the physician determined that she had lost her mother some months before and that her symptoms had begun not long after her mother's death.

The diagnosis: depression.

The happy outcome for both these people was relief of symptoms not by piecemeal treatment for the symptoms but by treatment directed at the depression that produced them.

They illustrate one aspect of depressive illness.

But there is another aspect illustrated by a woman who for fifteen years had been treated with antidepressant drugs and electroshock therapy for severe, sometimes suicidal, episodes of depression. Only when she was finally referred to the clinical research unit at the Western Psychiatric Institute and Clinic of the University of Pittsburgh School of Medicine was she found, after painstaking study, to have hyperparathyroidism. When the excessive gland function was treated, her depression improved.

In having a medical reason, a physical cause, for her seemingly psychiatric problem, she was no rare case at the Institute. There, Dr. David J. Kupfer, professor of psychiatry and director of the Institute, and his colleagues, studying depressed patients seriously enough affected to require hospitalization, have found 10 percent with underlying or concomitant medical diseases.

Other studies as well show that physical disorders—a rather lengthy list of them—can be the reason for what may seem to be purely psychologically induced depression. Failure to recognize those disorders when present can mean useless treatment, waste of time and money, or sometimes even worse.

The nightmare

Depression deserves a hard look and some basic understanding. It's a prime problem and often a confusing one, ranking as the most prevalent of psychic maladies, so widespread that it has been called the "common cold" of mental disturbances. The National Institute of Mental Health has estimated that as many as eight million Americans a year suffer depression severe enough to warrant treatment.

All of us, of course, have our ups and downs, days when we feel "low" and others when we feel on top of the world. Ordinary, everyday kinds of "lows" are brief and disappear spontaneously. Their possible causes are many, including the weather, a letdown after a holiday, insufficient sleep, excessive work demands and inadequate time to meet them.

But depression is another matter: no fleeting "down" feeling but rather a sustained, chronic change of mood, an extended lowering of the spirits. It can have behavioral and physical characteristics as well as emotional.

The mood is one of sadness, low feeling, blue feeling, despondency, gloominess, disgust, discouragement, or hopelessness. Once pleasurable activities—sports, games, hobbies—no longer are. Enjoyment of family and friends is reduced. A severely depressed person may become frightened at feeling that nothing and no one are important anymore.

On the behavioral side, there may be irritability, excessive response to small annoyances, difficulty in concentration, impairment of memory, loss of sexual interest, slowed or mixed-up thoughts, difficulties in getting started in the morning and in making decisions at any time, feelings of self-reproach or guilt. Anxiety may accompany depression, adding to the discomfort, making for nervousness so great that it often is impossible to sit or rest comfortably.

In addition, there may be physical symptoms: loss of appetite, weight loss, insomnia or restless sleep, headache, dizziness, indigestion, fatigue, weakness, sweating, coldness or tingling of hands or feet.

No one person has all these manifestations. Some people have relatively few but intense symptoms; others have a variety, somewhat milder in nature.

Masked depressions

One frequent source of confusion with psychologically induced depression lies in the physical symptoms. Depression has been called "the great masquerader" because although there may be mood and even behavioral changes, the physical symptoms often override.

Commonly, so great may be the concern with body discomforts that little attention is paid to the other indications of depression, or they may be thought to be results of physical symptoms. And, commonly, when medical help is sought, the patient details the physical complaints and fails to mention others.

Unless the patient is aware of the importance of the mood and behavioral disturbances, or, failing that, the physician is alert to the possibilities and makes an effort to ferret them out, there may be useless treatment for symptoms instead of cause.

Some studies have indicated that the elapsed time from onset of depression to its recognition ranges up to thirty-six months, during which patients often, if they receive any treatment, may be treated for other illnesses.

One recent study covered one hundred consecutive patients seen at the University of Mississippi Medical Center and the Jackson Veterans Administration Hospital, referred by physicians and found to be depressed. Many had seen their physicians on several occasions because of sleep disturbances, had asked specifically for sleeping pills, and, in almost 100 percent of the cases, had received them, with the depression overlooked. Many others had been treated with analgesics for aches and pains; some had received antacids; and still others had been given antinausea drugs. When carefully interviewed at the Center and the Hospital, they admitted to many other symptoms suggesting depression.

Effective treatment

When depression is psychologically based, when it is clearly recognized as such and any possible physical causes are excluded, treatment for it is commonly effective.

Many antidepressant medications are available. They include such agents as imipramine (trade named Tofranil), desipramine (trade named Norpramin), protriptyline (trade named Vivactil), nortriptyline (trade named Aventyl), doxepin (trade named Sinequan), and amitriptyline plus perphenazine (trade named Elavil and Etrafon).

Most antidepressants take about three weeks to begin to work and another few weeks before exerting their full effects. Side reactions to them are usually more annoying than serious. The most common are dryness of the mouth and some constipation. For the first few days there may be some sleepiness and occasionally a patient may feel a bit unusual or peculiar for a short time. When side reactions are troublesome, a switch may be made to another antidepressant which, in the individual case, may act against the depression with fewer, less bothersome, or no undesirable effects.

Once the symptoms of depression—including the physical—are gone, the antidepressant medication may be reduced gradually and then discontinued.

There is a kind of depressive illness called manic or bipolar in which recurrent bouts of severe depression alternate with episodes of great elation that in some cases may be manifested in flamboyant speech and action, or feelings of being unable to do anything wrong.

For manic-depressive illness, a relatively new drug, lithium carbonate, is often effective in preventing recurrences of both the mania and the depression.

But Now—to the Somatopsychic

What causes the depression?

A loss—the death of a loved one, a job loss, a financial setback, for example—may trigger it. And such a depression, which is brought on by an external event, is called *reactive* or *exogenous*.

Another kind, the *endogenous*, comes from within, from some internal event. Suddenly an individual may come to feel that he or she has failed in life. Although there may be no real (logical) grounds for this, nonetheless this is how the individual sees himself and becomes bereft of self-esteem and self-confidence. And now, matters that were once handled without difficulty—everyday affairs, family problems, social problems, financial problems—suddenly become monumental, too much to cope with.

Depression also can be mixed, both endogenous and exogenous. And some investigators believe that since many people suffer grief from a death in the family or other loss but, after a period of mourning, bounce back, there must be some internal, or endogenous, factor that is responsible in those who go into prolonged depression. Some investigators also believe that the unknown internal events that lead to endogenous depression may quite possibly be biochemical and may therefore involve a physical (biochemical) malfunctioning.

Aside from the latter possibility, depression can stem from clear-cut—or, more accurately, clearly defined—organic problems. The list of physical illnesses or disorders capable of producing many or all of the symptoms of depressive illness is sizable.

It includes infections such as hepatitis, mononucleosis, and influenza; hormonal (glandular) disorders such as those of the thyroid, parathyroid, and adrenal glands; malignancies, deficiency states, anemias, and other blood problems. It also includes reactions to the use of certain medications and, not uncommonly, to oral contraceptives.

And in all of these, not only may depression accompany or appear after the illness; it can sometimes be the very first manifestation.

Viral depressions

Among patients seeking help at a mental health clinic were an 18-year-old woman and a 23-year-old man. Both were suffering from depressed states. Yet the depression in the woman proved to be the result of infectious hepatitis; in the man, of infectious mononucleosis.

Both infectious hepatitis and infectious mononucleosis can take familiar forms.

Hepatitis, an infection of the liver, may strike suddenly

with fever (up to 102°), headache, muscle aches, general weakness, appetite loss, nausea at the sight of food, tender liver, and pain or pressure below the ribs on the right side. After a week or a little less, jaundice may appear (it doesn't always), and there may be vomiting, general body itching, darkening of urine, all persisting for two weeks or longer.

Mononucleosis, also known as glandular fever, may strike suddenly, too, with fever, headache, and sore throat, followed, after a few days, with painful swelling of under-the-jaw lymph nodes, sometimes also with swelling of lymph nodes under the arm and in the groin. Listlessness, weakness, and easy fatigability are common.

But both diseases can start insidiously and misleadingly with weakness, appetite loss, depressed mood, pessimism, and decreased ambition, and not infrequently the victims go first to a psychiatrist.

Both diseases are detectable by blood tests. And although there are no specific medications for them, they can be eased when properly diagnosed by medical measures.

The common cold, as we indicated earlier, is a viral illness that can produce gloominess while it lasts. Influenza has another kind of mental effect. Following a flu attack, many patients experience a period of worrisome weakness and depression that may persist as long as six weeks after all overt indications of the physical illness have disappeared. In one recent study carried out after a flu outbreak, one-fourth of the patients who were checked three weeks later reported depressed mood, pessimism, self-deprecation, diminished libido, appetite loss, sleep disturbance, and decreased ambition. Worrisome, indeed, if the source isn't recognized—and if there isn't a comforting awareness that all this, too, shall pass.

Endocrine gland disorders and depression

That endocrine disturbances can produce psychological disturbances will not be surprising when, in Chapter 8, we look closely at the system of glands, their key functions, and what happens with malfunctioning.

Here, with more detail to come later, just a brief indication of which endocrine disturbances can lead to depression.

We noted one earlier in this chapter in the case of the woman with long-overlooked hyperparathyroidism. It is no rarity for excessive secretions of the parathyroid glands to be manifested to begin with, and for long periods, by symptoms of depression alone.

Similarly, the first indication of adrenal gland disturbances can in some cases be depression, sometimes severe enough even to involve suicidal thoughts. That holds for Cushing's syndrome, in which there is overproduction of adrenal hormones. And it holds, too, for Addison's disease, in which the glands are underactive rather than overactive. Both diseases, when properly diagnosed, are medically treatable.

Among the most common endocrine causes of mental and emotional disturbances are thyroid gland disorders. Hypothyroidism, or underfunctioning, is typically associated with depressed mood, pessimism, and poor self-esteem. It is readily correctable if suspected and diagnosed, yet often it goes unsuspected for long periods. It can give rise to other behavioral problems as well. So can the opposite condition, hyperthyroidism, in which the gland is too active. And we will be devoting considerable attention to the thyroid in Chapter 8.

The Pill

Since the advent of oral contraceptives in the 1950's, a wide range of side effects has been reported, each with a flurry of publicity.

Attention has been paid to increased risk of strokes and coronary thrombosis (heart attack), high blood pressure, migraine headaches, aggravation of existing varicose veins, and elevation of blood fats. (It should be stressed that the more serious side effects are uncommon; nonetheless, they indicate the need for regular medical supervision and checking.)

Although less well known, mental depression is one of the most common side effects, occurring in as many as 5 percent of women.

Why should oral contraceptives produce depression?

There is evidence that mood is affected by the concentrations of specific chemicals, the amines, in certain parts of the brain. Depressive illness has been associated with low levels of these amines, particularly one called norepinephrine. Norepinephrine is produced from two compounds, tyrosine and another with a jawbreaking name, 5-hydroxytryptamine, which is made from still another compound, tryptophan. Oral contraceptives have been found to alter the body's handling of both tyrosine and tryptophan. And it seems likely that the alteration occurs because in some women the Pill leads to a deficiency of vitamin B_6, or pyridoxine, which is needed for the proper handling of these compounds.

Dr. Frank Winston, a physician with considerable experience with Pill-induced depression, first described the beneficial effect of administering large doses of pyridoxine. Later, other investigators, including a group at St. Mary's Hospital, London, headed by Professor Victor Wynn, carried out careful trials that showed satisfactory responses in women in whom tests revealed evidence of vitamin B_6 deficiency.

The doses used to overcome the deficiency and the depression are large. In the London study, 20 milligrams of B_6 was given twice a day, an amount equal to about twenty times, all told, what a normal, healthy adult needs to take in through food.

Provided a woman who is suffering from depressed feelings induced by an oral contraceptive is aware of the possible relationship, or seeks help from a physician who considers the possibility, treatment with B_6 may offer help.

Another alternative may be switching to another oral contraceptive since different brands do have different kinds and amounts of ingredients. And still another choice, of course, is switching to a different method of contraception.

Deficiency states

Vitamin B_6 deficiency, induced in some women by oral contraceptives, is only one example of deficiency states that may produce depression.

Deficiency of folic acid, another of the B vitamins, can do the same. It can also produce puzzling fatigue and other disturbances. And as we'll see later in this book, the deficiency, which is readily correctable, is by no means rare.

Deficiency of another B vitamin, niacin, can, when severe, lead to pellagra. And although pellagra is not as common as it once was, it still does occur in the United States, particularly in the southeastern part of the country. It should not occur with a well-balanced diet; the vitamin is present in liver, whole-grain cereals, lean meats, fish, fowl, peanuts, milk, potatoes, and leafy vegetables. But for one reason or another—fad diets, for example, as well as finances—not all people consume a well-balanced diet.

Niacin is essential for many purposes in the body, including the well-being of the nervous system. And when deficiency leads toward pellagra, there can be psychological as well as physical effects.

Among early symptoms are weakness and loss of appetite and weight. Later, there may be headaches, gastrointestinal disturbances, and skin spots. And among the psychological signs may be memory impairment, insomnia, irrational behavior, irritability, and depression.

The deficiency, of course, is correctable with administration of niacin in divided daily doses that may range from 300 to 1,000 milligrams and with correction of diet.

Blood disorders

Among patients found in one recent study to be seeking psychiatric help when what they really needed was medical aid were a 56-year-old woman with depression that proved to be the result of pernicious anemia and a 50-year-old man whose depression was caused by a blood problem called polycythemia vera. Both responded to treatment for their underlying problem; it is highly unlikely they would have been much helped by antidepressant medication or the most extended psychotherapy.

These are two more physical problems that can sometimes be manifested first, as they were in these cases, by depression.

Pernicious anemia is a special kind of anemia. It involves a deficiency of a vitamin—B_{12}. But the deficiency is not the result of lack of adequate dietary intake. Instead, the vitamin cannot be absorbed because of inadequate amounts or complete lack of a factor in the stomach needed for its absorption. This can be overcome readily, and we'll be looking at pernicious anemia in more detail, along with other anemias that can have behavioral effects, in Chapter 7.

Polycythemia vera in a way is the opposite of anemia. Where commonly in anemia there is a shortage of red cells in the blood, in polycythemia there are too many. The disease has its greatest incidence in middle and late life and in men, although it can occur earlier and in women as well.

The disease develops slowly and the onset of symptoms is gradual. There may be headache, lassitude, dizziness. Visual disturbances, itching, and burning and tingling sensations are often experienced. Shortness of breath may develop and there may be bluish-redness of the skin of the face and extremities.

But in some cases depression may appear before any other indications of polycythemia.

Proper diagnosis, made with the help of blood tests, is important and not only to avoid needless treatment of depression. If uncontrolled, the excessive number of red cells and the consequent thickening of blood can lead to artery blockage and heart attack or stroke.

Treatment is aimed at reducing the red cell numbers and blood viscosity. Venesection, or bloodletting, is often used and may be done at first once or twice a week, later every three or four months. In some cases, in addition to or instead of venesection, injections of radiophosphorus may be given to help reduce the overproduction of red cells. Sometimes, drugs such as busulfan or melphalan may be of value. With vigorous treatment, polycythemia is controllable.

Other organic diseases causing depression

Some years ago, a distinguished psychiatrist, Dr. Z. J. Lipowski of McGill University, reported having three patients referred to him over a brief period, each with a diagnosis of severe depression. In each case, Lipowski discovered, the depression was the result of undetected cancer of the pancreas.

Other cancers—of the stomach and other abdominal organs—have been found to produce a curious depressive syndrome. Victims suffer from fatigue, loss of normal ambitions and interests, depressed mood, and premonitions of doom—at a time when the tumors are otherwise silent.

One form of cancer of the lung—oat cell—has recently been reported to sometimes manifest itself first as depression. And accurate diagnosis of the cancer without delay has become even more important than ever because of recent promising results in the treatment of this kind of lung malignancy.

Also reported recently, a case of depression in a 46-year-old man that proved to be due to high blood pressure and disappeared when the pressure was lowered by treatment.

Drug-induced depressions

No less than possible physical causes, drugs need to be considered as possible factors before depression is categorized as psychological.

As side effects, many drugs can produce emotional and behavioral as well as physical disturbances and we will discuss these more fully in Chapter 17.

Here we can look briefly at some of the agents capable of sometimes provoking depressive reactions.

One of the most striking examples is reserpine, which is often used in the treatment of high blood pressure. As many as 15 percent of patients receiving the drug have been reported to experience depressive phenomena. Usually, the depression lifts when the connection with reserpine is recognized and the drug is abandoned in favor of another antihypertensive agent.

But it's important to remember that reserpine is available for use not only by itself but also as an ingredient in many combination drugs with different brand names and sometimes not only a patient but his physician may be unaware of this. Among combination drugs incorporating reserpine are Butiserpazide, Diupres, Diutensen-R, Dralserp, Exna-R, Hydromox-R, Hydropres, Hydroserpine, Hydrotensin, Metatensin, Naquival, Rau-Sed, Regroton, Renese-R, Ruhexatal, Salutensin, Sandril, Ser-Ap-Es, Serpasil, Serpasil-Apresoline, and Serpasil-Esidrix.

Alphamethyldopa, trade named Aldomet, which is also used in the treatment of high blood pressure, can also trigger mild depression. And other drugs, particularly minor tranquilizers such as Valium, may have a depressive effect on some patients.

SEE ALSO: If you suffer from depressive symptoms, or, in fact, from any of a number of other seemingly psychosomatic problems such as fatigue, tension, irritability, anxiety, it is possible that Chapters 4 and 6 may give you a clue. Caffeinism has been found recently to be a not uncommon problem capable of producing such symptoms, and if you can relate your problem to caffeinism as described in Chapter 6, you may be able to solve it on your own and quite readily. Cerebral allergy, too, in the view of a small but growing group of investigators, is capable of triggering such symptoms, and cerebral allergy is described in detail in Chapter 11.

A sleep test for depression

With a willingness to consider that what appears to be a psychologically induced depression may in fact be one with a physical base instead and with a vigorous effort to seek out a possible organic cause, a knowledgeable physician often may discover the true cause. Even well-informed patients may sometimes be able to suspect where the problem lies.

But there remain situations in which it would be helpful to have some objective test for distinguishing depression caused by medical disease.

Such a test has been developed by Dr. David J. Kupfer and his associates at the Western Psychiatric Institute and Clinic and is based on the character of the rapid eye movement (REM) stage of sleep.

Sleep is not a one-stage process but rather one of several stages. In one of these, REM, the brain is more active, dreaming occurs, and there are bursts of rapid eye movements. In normal people, REM begins about ninety minutes after the onset of sleep.

In one of their first studies, Dr. Kupfer and his team were able to determine that in people with primary depression, unrelated to any physical problem, REM occurs much sooner than the normal ninety minutes; and the more severe the depression, the sooner REM develops.

The Pittsburgh team then went on to study two groups of patients. All were depressed, but in one group the patients had physical illnesses that had not been detected before they were admitted to the Western Psychiatric Institute. This group included patients with depression associated with hypothyroidism, hyperthyroidism, viral infection, cancer, and other medical problems.

Between the two groups, the depressive symptoms were

indistinguishable. Not so, however, the character of REM sleep.

In both groups, REM sleep appeared earlier than in normal people. But in the depressed group without medical problems, it appeared much earlier, average time forty-two minutes, while in the group with medical problems, the average time was seventy-three minutes.

There were other differences. Total REM time averaged seventy-four minutes for the first group, forty-four minutes for the second. In addition, total REM activity (the number of eye movements) proved to be more than three times greater among the depressed without medical illness, and for them, too, the REM density (the ratio of total REM activity to total REM time) was twice as great.

Thus, the sleep test can be a valuable tool, when there is any doubt, in determining whether a depression is associated with medical illness or not. It promises to prevent the inappropriate use of antidepressant drugs or electroshock therapy in patients with medical diseases causing depression, treatments, at best, wasteful and sometimes dangerous in that they may allow a medical condition to progress beyond the curable stage.

It promises to have other values as well. For one thing, the finding of REM characteristics indicative of primary depression in older people with severe confusion and other behavioral disturbance could avoid a possible hasty diagnosis of hopeless senility and point to the fact that primary depression is present and should be treated vigorously.

Moreover, the test can be used when psychologically induced depression is present to determine within a few days whether a particular patient will or will not respond to a particular drug, whereas otherwise it usually takes several weeks for effects of antidepressants to be observable. The Pittsburgh team has found that after only two days of drug treatment, patients who will respond well to the drug already show desirable changes in REM characteristics to a much greater degree than the poor responders.

The sleep test can be carried out in a sleep clinic. And sleep clinics are being set up at more and more university hospitals and major medical centers. If you suffer from depression and your physician can't determine with certainty whether there may be a medical reason for it or not, you may benefit from referral to a clinic. If you have difficulty finding a nearby clinic, the address of one can be obtained from The American Association of Sleep Disorders Centers, University of Cincinnati Sleep Disorder Center, Christian R. Holmes Hospital, Eden and Bethesda Avenues, Cincinnati, Ohio 45219.

4. When Anxiety Has a Physical Base

She was 25 years old, an apparent victim of severe anxiety that would require psychiatric help. She had been experiencing episodes of great apprehension. Often these were accompanied by sweats, vomiting, and diarrhea.

But her real problem proved to be a heart rhythm disturbance, paroxysmal atrial tachycardia, during which the heartbeat rate may shoot up to one hundred or more beats a minute.

Although it may be associated with heart disease, the racing heart can also occur in the absence of disease and in relatively young people. Suddenly, the role of the pacemaker, an area of heart tissue that normally sets the beat rate, is taken over temporarily by another area. An episode may last minutes, hours, sometimes days, ending as abruptly as it began.

When the young woman received quinidine, a drug with a normalizing effect on some heart rhythm disturbances, the tachycardia and the anxiety attacks stopped.

It may seem almost incredible but in another instance the reason for anxiety proved to be scabies; and when the mite infestation was diagnosed and treated, the anxiety, which in this case had been the first manifestation, preceding the itching of scabies, disappeared.*

Nor are these by any means the only physical disorders which can lead to anxiety that seems psychogenic in origin and that may be the first manifestation and may mask the real problem.

---

* *It's not incredible at all. Scabies is a problem widely misunderstood by many physicians as well as the public.*

It was scabies that accounted for an incident involving a psychiatrist and a child he was treating for what was presumed to be emotionally induced eczema. But the child's itching skin problem did not abate; and when, in desperation, the psychiatrist took the child to a dermatology clinic, he was shocked to be told that the problem was scabies. To add to his discomfiture, he himself had developed an itching eruption that he had attributed to his own inner rage at the boy's "hostility," and that, too, proved to be scabies, which, like the boy's, responded to brief treatment.

Scabies recently has reached epidemic proportions in the United States. Yet many cases escape recognition because of a generally low index of suspicion.

For one thing, a common notion has been that scabies is no longer a problem in this country. One medical dictionary published in 1966 described it as "an eruption almost extinct in the United States." Also, the disease is looked upon as limited to the poor, overcrowded, and nonfastidious, when, in fact, it affects the wealthy and scrupulously clean as well.

Scabies can be acquired through contact with an affected individual or with clothing, bed linen, or towels contaminated by mites or their eggs or larvae. Nor is close contact required. Up to 16 percent of scabies cases result from dancing or holding hands, and even a quick handshake can transmit the mite.

Once on the skin, the tiny female mite burrows under the surface to lay eggs, leaving a wavy line not always visible to the naked eye. In her four- to five-week life, she lays one or two eggs daily, which, after three to five days, hatch into larvae. Five days to two weeks later, the young develop into adults, mate, and the females dig new burrows.

Scabies can produce intense itching, worse at night after the bed has been warmed by body heat. Wheals (hives) may develop over the entire body as an allergic reaction to the parasites or their excretions.

Diagnosis can be made with the aid of a hand lens that reveals the characteristic scabies burrows. Treatment is relatively simple: application of a cream or lotion containing gamma benzene hexachloride (Kwell) over the entire body below the chin, washed off after twenty-four hours. Often this is all that is required. If necessary, a second application can be used.

Anxiety defined

Anxiety is a common enough problem. Yet even though ours has been called the Age of Anxiety, and scores of millions of prescriptions for tranquilizers to ease it are written each year, anxiety is not easy to define precisely.

A usual definition of anxiety is "tension or uneasiness from the anticipation of danger, the source of which is largely unknown or unrecognized." It is distinguished from fear, which is an emotional response to a recognized and usually external threat or danger.

Almost all of us have some familiarity with anxiety. Anxious feelings are common among students taking examinations and among patients waiting to see physicians. An interview for a job is apt to cause anxiety, and it is felt if one hears that a family member or a friend has had an accident or has been admitted to a hospital. These are simple, event-related instances of "normal" anxiety. The anxious feelings usually disappear shortly after the event.

But chronic anxiety is another matter.

Anxiety symptoms

With chronic anxiety, the victim may be suffused with unpleasant feelings of tension, dread, or impending doom, and may be unable to think clearly, reason logically, show good judgment, or remember accurately.

In response to this state, physical symptoms occur and may be alarming enough to cause the anxiety to spiral.

Commonly, there are heart and respiratory symptoms: palpitations (heartbeats that are unusually rapid, strong, or irregular enough to intrude upon consciousness) and breathlessness.

Some anxious patients develop gastrointestinal symptoms: abdominal cramps, nausea, vomiting, and diarrhea. Other frequent complaints include headache, backache, chest pain or "tightness," fatigue, weakness, insomnia, increased perspiration, and dry mouth.

In some cases, there are episodes of acute anxiety—attacks of panic or unbearable apprehension, racing pulse, rapid breathing, profuse perspiration, and tremors.

Nonphysical causes

A major source of anxiety, in the view of many psychiatrists, is man's conscience, an internal censor that begins to develop early in life in response to real or assumed attitudes of parents and others close to the child. As the child grows, he may accept some of these standards, reject some, and thus eventually develop his own system of right and wrong. When this system, or conscience, or internal censor, clashes with the individual's natural desires in some situations (for possession, love, sex, vengeance), his personality is in a sense divided and he may experience feelings of apprehension and inner restlessness.

There are other sources. The conscience may take over the approval-disapproval functions of parents, teachers, and others. But the individual still has need for the approval of others. And anxiety may arise not only from a conflict with conscience but also because of the disapproval, or fear of disapproval, of other people—family, friends, employer.

Anxiety also can be based on current problems that cause uncertainty, frustration, and stress because of an inability to find solutions to them, problems such as an unsatisfactory job, an undisciplined or difficult child, economic difficulty, an unhappy marriage.

Some hold that ours is an Age of Anxiety because we have generally more stress and grounds for anxiety than did people before us. They point to a lengthy list of turmoils, including ideological conflicts, hot and cold wars, the atom bomb, technological speedup, fantastic expansion of human mobility, problems of population, poverty, pollution, and race, and changes in sex and marriage customs, family relations, and the whole spectrum of moral attitudes.

Others believe, however, that while we have such

grounds for anxiety, preceding populations had their own assortment.

In any case, anxiety—excessive and stress-induced or emotionally induced—is very much with us.

Treatment

Are antianxiety drugs—tranquilizers—necessary?

They have a place, but they are not inevitably the answer. If there is no question that tranquilizers have revolutionized psychiatry, there also seems to be no question that not enough people require mood-affecting drugs to justify the 178,000,000 prescriptions written for them in this country in one year.

Perhaps one concerned physician is right. He asks these questions: "How do physicians acquire such unquestioning faith in drugs? Are they stampeded by their patients? Because they serve a public that has been brainwashed to think that there is a 'pill for every ill,' do they believe the patient will be disappointed if he doesn't receive something tangible in return for sharing his problems?"

But he answers thus: "Many physicians feel ill-equipped to deal with the emotional aspects of a patient's illness and are unwilling to embroil themselves in a lengthy and financially unrewarding discussion with him. No doubt a pill is the easy way out."

Tranquilizers, of course, don't cure anxiety. They can relieve the symptoms and they can be valuable for that purpose when anxiety interferes with job and other aspects of daily living.

But a patient with anxiety often can benefit from simple counseling. Often he is unable to relate his anxiety to his job, marital, or other problems. There may be an assumption that the anxiety comes from some unknown source over which he has no control. Often problem identification alone—with the help of any physician who takes the time for it—can provide a considerable measure of relief. After that, if the problem cannot be handled by the patient alone, expert help—perhaps from a psychiatrist or not infrequently from a marital, vocational, or other counselor—is called for.

There are also behavioral techniques that often can be effective in handling anxiety. Some knowledgeable physicians teach anxious patients to relax in a systematic way. Some teach patients systematic desensitization. Both are relatively simple to learn.

For example, one method of relaxation starts with taking time out to sit down and for five minutes or so just try to relax mentally and physically. If you feel tension anywhere in your body, try to let it go, making yourself as limp as a rag doll.

Then, take an additional few minutes for one or more simple exercises, done slowly, smoothly, without jerking. Seated comfortably, raise your arms slowly overhead, then let them drop. Do the same with your legs. After each drop, pause a few seconds to appreciate the relaxed effect. Breathe deeply, exhale slowly.

Lie on your back on the floor. Close your eyes. Take a deep breath. Exhale slowly. Tighten all the muscles in your body. Then let go. Breathe deeply, exhale slowly.

Still on the floor, shrug your shoulders up to your ears and then let them fall back. Turn your head far to the left, then to the front, and relax. Repeat to the right. Breathe deeply and exhale after each movement.

Another simple systematic relaxation technique that has been reported to work for many in moderating anxiety involves three steps. First, sit comfortably, feet on floor, eyes closed, and let breathing become relaxed, with air gently flowing in and out of your lungs, after which muscles can be readily allowed to relax. As a second step, relax your mind, letting it drift naturally and gently to some pleasant, relaxing, restful memory. Usually this can be achieved within a minute. Then, in the third step, present the memory gently to your mind. Allow yourself to be there, to experience the memory. Don't concentrate. If your mind wanders off, simply bring yourself back, gently, to presenting the memory to your mind again.

Systematic desensitization is somewhat akin to desensitization to allergies. In the latter, when a particular pollen or other material is found to cause hay fever or other allergic manifestation, an extract of the material is injected, at first in the tiniest of doses but then, gradually, in increasing amounts. The idea is to build tolerance to the material so it no longer causes trouble.

Desensitization for anxiety starts with relaxation such as that which can be achieved with the three-step method. Then, while relaxed, you create visual images in which you imagine yourself in a series of anxiety-evoking situations while remaining relaxed. You start with the mildly bothersome situations and work up gradually to the more threatening.

The theory is that when anxiety-arousing situations can be faced comfortably in fantasy, there will be a carry-over into the real world. And, in fact, desensitization has been reported to work often, even in cases of severe phobias.

Somatopsychic Anxiety

The young woman with a heart rhythm disturbance and the patient with scabies represent, as we noted earlier, only two examples of physically induced anxiety.

Many other physical diseases or disorders not only can be accompanied by anxiety but may be first manifested by anxiety symptoms, later to be followed by others.

Tumor-provoked anxiety

Although anxiety as a first indication of a growth is not very common, it is of course important to note that it can occur.

Cancer of the pancreas, as we noted in the preceding chapter, sometimes may trigger severe depression. Alternatively, sometimes it may provoke anxiety. Later, other symptoms appear. There may be abdominal pain, variable in nature and often radiating to the back, which may be relieved by sitting up and bending forward. Other symptoms may include jaundice, weight loss, appetite loss, nausea, vomiting, and constipation.

Brain tumor—fortunately, not a common disease; in fact, classifiable as a rare one—does not, contrary to general belief, invariably produce headache as a first symptom. Anxiety may come first. Or, often, there may be slow, progressive disturbances in balance, sight, or smell, or unexplained weakness in arm and leg muscles. Often, when headaches first appear, they do so in the morning and are brief. Later they may become very severe and constant, although not invariably. Other symptoms may include persistent nausea and vomiting, lethargy, drowsiness, and impairment of mental function.

Some cancers of the ovary may sometimes be first manifested by anxiety. Other early symptoms are vague lower abdominal discomfort and mild digestive complaints. Later, as the ovary enlarges, the abdomen may become swollen and there may be pelvic pain.

A carcinoid is a yellow circumscribed tumor that may occur in the small intestine or elsewhere in the gastrointestinal tract. In some cases, anxiety may be the first symptom, although more commonly the earliest manifestation is flushing of the skin triggered by food, alcohol, or emotion. Abdominal discomfort with recurrent diarrhea develops. A few patients experience asthmatic wheezing.

A pheochromocytoma is a small tumor of an adrenal gland. It is relatively rare, much more often benign than malignant. But it can secrete excessive amounts of two adrenal hormones, epinephrine (adrenaline) and norepinephrine. It may provoke anxiety first. Other symptoms can include severe headache, sweating, palpitation, visual blurring, flushing of the face, tremulousness, and nausea and vomiting. A pheochromocytoma is a rare cause of high blood pressure.

All of these diseases often can be treated effectively when diagnosed without excessive delay through careful physical examination and laboratory and other tests.

Endocrine gland disorders

Endocrine disturbances can and frequently do have emotional and behavioral effects, as we noted in the preceding chapter on depression and as we'll see in detail in Chapter 8.

And among the gland disorders, some that can produce depression as a first manifestation in some cases can be responsible for anxiety as a first manifestation in others. This is true of hypothyroidism, or underfunctioning of the thyroid gland; hyperparathyroidism, or overfunctioning of the parathyroids; and adrenal gland overfunctioning, as in Cushing's syndrome.

In addition, hyperthyroidism, or overfunctioning of the thyroid, can sometimes be responsible for anxiety and, beyond this, for other emotional and behavioral as well as various physical symptoms.

Diabetes, too, as we will see in Chapter 8, can be an insidious problem, and anxiety sometimes can be a first manifestation.

Heart and blood vessel (cardiovascular) disorders

At least in a few cases, patients with cardiovascular disorders may first seek help for anxiety.

Cerebral atherosclerosis—in which the inner linings of brain arteries thicken because of fatty accumulations—can, of course, when it advances to the point of choking off circulation to a portion of the brain, produce a stroke. But, short of this, without complete choking off, the deposits may interfere enough with blood flow to produce forgetfulness, confusion, and personality changes, with anxiety sometimes being the first manifestation.

Detection of cerebral atherosclerosis—and there are X-ray and other means for achieving this—is important because in some cases surgery to bypass narrowed vessels can be effective and in some other cases, as we'll see in Chapter 15, medical measures can help.

That's also true when atherosclerosis affects the coronary arteries feeding the heart muscle. Here again, in some cases, anxiety may be the first manifestation. More commonly, of course, coronary atherosclerosis produces angina pectoris, the crushing chest pain on effort. Treatment for the coronary disease and its effects—with medication or, when essential, bypass surgery—often can be effective.

Hypoglycemia (low blood sugar), epilepsy, caffeinism, cerebral allergy

All of the above problems may sometimes provoke anxiety. They may also be linked with other behavioral and emotional disturbances, and you will find them discussed in some detail later, each in a separate chapter.

Drug-induced anxiety

Drug-induced anxiety is not, by any means, rare.

Anxiety can be provoked by cocaine. It also can stem from amphetamines. Used widely, and often illegally, by drivers to keep awake, students to do the same in preparation for exams, and by those who become "hooked," or dependent, on them, amphetamines and amphetaminelike compounds also are often used in weight reducing. They include such preparations, all supposed to be available on prescription only, as Benzedrine, Biphetamine, Obetrol, Fetamin, Delcobese, and Pondimin. Tenuate, another commonly used appetite-suppressing drug, also can produce anxiety in some people.

Anxiety also can occur as a drug-withdrawal effect when use of barbiturates, tranquilizers, or alcohol is stopped.

Some drugs, such as Drixoral, used for nasal congestion,

also can have anxiety as a side effect for some people, and this is also true of barbiturates (sleeping pills) and antihistamines used for allergy.

And the list of agents capable of causing anxiety as a side reaction in some cases goes on. It includes a number of compounds used for lowering high blood pressure, among them, Apresoline, Hydropres, Rauzide, Reserpine, Salutensin, and Ser-Ap-Es.

Also included are some drugs used to combat depression, such as Elavil and Tofranil. Also, paradoxically, Valium, even though it may be used to combat anxiety, and Etrafon and Triavil, two agents that are often used for anxiety and depression.

5. *Psychogenic Fatigue— or Is It?*

Not long ago, a 44-year-old woman was admitted to a Canadian hospital with a three-year history of continuous fatigue. She also complained of leg numbness, dizziness, blurred vision, daily headaches, and constipation.

But fatigue was her major concern. It had become extreme in the last two years, had made housework and care of her two children impossible.

She was also clearly anxious and depressed and her problems could easily have seemed to be due to emotional disturbance.

Yet the real reason for them became evident after a thorough study. On physical examination, the only abnormalities that could be found were neurological, or nerve-related. They included some loss of sensation below the knees and slight weakness of the legs. Among the various tests that were then performed were blood and spinal fluid measurements, which indicated one abnormal reading: low levels of a B vitamin, folic acid.

By the sixth day after she was started on folic acid treatment, the blood picture showed some improvement; by day ten, there was further improvement and she was discharged from the hospital, though continuing on folic acid. Two months later, she was a different woman. Her fatigue was gone; her depression and anxiety had vanished; she had no constipation; her headaches had become occasional.

Although folic acid is an essential vitamin, a deficiency of it has generally not been believed to produce neurologic symptoms. The finding that it can produce such symptoms and can give rise to severe fatigue—made at the Clinical Research Institute and the Hôtel-Dieu Hospital, Montreal, where the woman and several other patients with similar symptoms responded to folic acid treatment—is important because folic acid deficiency, as we'll see in Chapter 7, is common.

Undue fatigue has many possible causes. It can be psychogenic. But it can also stem from physical disturbances, some of them disease states, some of them not.

Normal fatigue

Normal fatigue has been described in many ways.

It has, for example, been called a "negative appetite for activity" which may be more pronounced for the specific kind of activity that has produced it and may even sometimes be absent for other kinds of activity.

As one medical dictionary defines it, it is "that state following a period of mental or bodily activity characterized by a lessened capacity for work and reduced efficiency of accomplishment, usually accompanied by a feeling of weariness, sleepiness, or irritability; it may also supervene when from any cause energy expenditure outstrips restorative processes, e.g., lack of sleep or food."

Dr. Ernest L. Hartmann, a distinguished Boston psychiatrist and sleep investigator, points out that there are two basic kinds of normal fatigue or tiredness that affect all of us.

One, coming after a day of purely physical activity such as skiing or manual labor, is "simple" or "physical" tiredness. Such tiredness is usually associated with a relaxed feeling in the muscles, even the facial and head muscles, and very seldom with any tightness or headaches. In fact, simple, physical tiredness is usually considered pleasant or neutral, unassociated with any characteristic psychic changes.

The other, "mental" tiredness, often develops after a long day of intellectually or emotionally demanding work. "This tiredness, with which most of us are all too familiar," says Dr. Hartmann, "is often accompanied by tension or tightness of the muscles, especially the muscles of the face and head; and it is usually described with a negative tone—it is unpleasant, or, at best, neutral. It sometimes has the paradoxical effect of making it hard to fall asleep."

Certainly, physical fatigue brought on by hard work or play provokes no alarm; we know we'll recover energy with rest. And while mental fatigue may have some unpleasant aspects, we know, too, that it is a temporary matter.

Chronic fatigue, however, is of considerable concern. There have been reports from some physicians that as many as half of their patients have excessive tiredness as at least one complaint. And persistent tiredness fuels an industry very successful at selling nostrums for "tired blood." It also occasions much doctor-shopping and complaints that "nothing seems to help."

Psychological fatigue

"I have yet to find," one physician has observed, "a young housewife with a mother-in-law in her kitchen who is not tired. And a workingman who is frustrated by his boss may hardly have the strength to get out of bed each morning."

Possible psychological causes for fatigue are many. A chronic fatigue state, as we've seen earlier, may accompany depression or anxiety. And no pep pill, tonic, iron preparation, or vitamin booster will make any real dent in the fatigue until the depression or anxiety is overcome.

Short of depression or anxiety, unhappiness can foster fatigue. And the fatigue won't depart until the unhappiness is resolved. That may call for taking time to sit down and review the particular life situation and pinpoint, if possible, the cause of unhappiness—perhaps difficulties with spouse and/or children. Such difficulties may be ameliorated a little by a talk with them about the unhappiness; at least communication will be improved. In some cases, professional help—from a marital or other counselor, physician, or psychiatrist—may be needed to figure out how to handle the difficulties.

Indecision can cause fatigue. "Ambivalence on any type of decision-making is exhausting," says Dr. Richard Kohl, professor of psychiatry at Cornell Medical Center, New York City. "You must recognize the source of conflict and try to deal with and resolve it in a sensible way, realizing that some chance has to be taken. The very process of decision-making is taking a chance, and a wrong decision can sometimes be better than no decision at all."

The not inconsequential boredom problem

"Sooner or later, it happens to most of us. You wake one morning, it is February in your soul, the tide is out, and nothing is visible except mud flats. There isn't much pain, just a great emptiness. The excitement of living has ebbed away, leaving only a littered line of memories along the shore to mark the receding tide of passion. You go through the day by rote, doing what you should do, more like a spectator than an actor. The condition is so common most languages have a world for it. For the Romans it was *taedium;* for the French it is *ennui;* for Americans it's boredom, the blues, the blahs, or, when it becomes serious, depression." So observed Dr. Sam Keen, writing recently in *Psychology Today.*

Boredom with the daily routine doesn't necessarily come on that dramatically nor become serious enough to produce depression. But it is a not uncommon cause of chronic fatigue, and studies in neurophysiology have provided some insight into why.

Investigators have been able to locate specific brain structures in animals, stimulate them with small electrical currents, and show that some of these structures have an inhibitory effect while others constitute an activating system.

Mood and ability to perform at any given time depend on the degree of activity of the two systems. When the inhibitory system is dominant, the individual is in a state of fatigue. When the activating system is in the ascendancy, he is ready to increase performance.

The existence of the two systems helps to explain some previously puzzling phenomena. For example, everyone has had the experience of feeling physically or mentally fatigued only to find that when something unexpected happens—perhaps good news or bad, or a sudden inspiration—the fatigue disappears. What has happened is that the activating system has been stimulated by the unexpected and has attained dominance over the inhibitory system.

Even after a good night's sleep and only a few hours of work, not enough to cause physical fatigue, we may become mentally fatigued and bored if the surroundings are monotonous and the work is dull. Then the activating system is dampened and the inhibitory one becomes dominant.

Monotony involves sameness. Even the most interesting, challenging, thought-provoking job can become monotonous if it goes on day after day, or even hour after hour, without change of pace.

When fatigue stems from monotony and boredom, some relatively simple measures can be valuable. They include efforts to vary the daily round as much as feasible, to seek new and more active ways to spend leisure time, perhaps to revive old interests that have been neglected. At work, as much as possible, it can be helpful to switch from one activity to another (if that is in the nature of the work) every so often, to take brief breaks, to pause and get up from a desk job and walk about even if for no more than a few steps. Lessening the fatigue stress of monotony may well increase efficiency of performance.

The horsepower problem

That sedentary living, with insufficient physical activity, can be a cause of chronic fatigue should be no surprise. Yet it is a cause that can be overlooked while a search for more exotic reasons is pursued.

According to some estimates, the human body with maximum effort is capable of generating as much as 14 horsepower. At rest, it generates only 0.1 horsepower. And many who live sedentary lives may rarely call upon it to generate more. They may experience, for lack of use, some degree of muscular atrophy, or wasting, becoming undermuscled for their weight and lacking sufficient endurance even for sedentary work. It has been suggested, too, that in some cases, the unused horsepower goes into building tensions that become a factor in producing fatigue and sometimes other complaints as well.

Many cases have been reported like that of a man in his late thirties who had progressed well in his profession and should have been at the height of his capacity. Instead, he began to experience fatigue. The fatigue became chronic. Along with it, he suffered from sleeping difficulty and increasing difficulty in concentrating. He could handle his work, but only with great effort.

A knowledgeable physician, after thorough examination, recognized where the trouble might lie and prescribed a program of activity, of regular exercise, beginning easily and progressing gradually. Within a few months, there was a marked change. Activity proved reinvigorating.

Dr. Kenneth Cooper, who began research into physical conditioning while a military physician associated with the astronaut program and went on in civilian life to develop an aerobics system to help in achieving conditioning, treats women as well as men. "One of the major complaints I hear from patients," he told an interviewer, "is, 'Doctor, I'm always tired.' These are women in apparently good health who are already exhausted at 10 in the morning. We find that they are so poorly conditioned—their endurance levels are so low—that they would qualify at the lowest point on the aerobics fitness chart."

The President's Council on Physical Fitness has defined physical fitness, in fact, as "the ability to bear up, to withstand stress, and to persevere under difficult circumstances where an unfit person would quit!"

And when the American Aerospace Medical Association did a study on the "Medical Aspects of Aircraft Pilot Fatigue," it concluded that among the steps that needed to be taken to prevent flight fatigue, "First and foremost is the maintenance of one's physical fitness by regular periods of exercise."

Food and fatigue

Recently, a group of investigators headed by Dr. Samuel J. Arnold of Morristown, New Jersey, reported a generally unsuspected factor in some, perhaps a goodly number of, cases of fatigue. It appears that what you eat or fail to eat for breakfast can have considerable bearing.

Studying 138 generally healthy men and women, the investigators found that 79 percent either skipped breakfast or slighted it, eating at best juice, cereal, bread, and coffee, and getting little protein.

Forty-nine of the breakfast slighters experienced fatigue or what had been puzzling fluid retention or both. They undertook to try including in the first meal of the day either the whites of four or five eggs, or fish, meat, or cheese (mozzarella, cottage, or provalone), or artificially flavored gelatins (proteins) with at least two tablespoons of brewer's yeast. They also reduced sugar and bread intake.

Forty-seven of the forty-nine experienced clear-cut, and in some cases dramatic, reductions in fatigue and fluid retention. And, considering the results, the investigators urged physicians to determine what patients have for breakfast and, where necessary, to make modifications before undertaking to prescribe energizers or implicate psyches.

If a change in the breakfast menu can help some fatigue sufferers, others may benefit from eating four, five, or six smaller meals a day. Eating at spaced intervals in this way often can do more to maintain energy levels than eating the same amount of food in three meals a day.

Dieting for weight reduction can be a cause of fatigue.

The fact is that with weight problems of concern to upward of forty million Americans—and some estimates go far higher—at any moment some twenty million people in this country are on some kind of reducing diet.

Very commonly, because there is great preoccupation with fast loss, the diet is a fad diet. Dieting has been called our number one national pastime.

Among the bizarre diets that come and go in fashion are magic-pair diets: lamb chops and grapefruit, eggs and spinach, or bananas and skim milk, and infinite variations on the theme that somehow two-food combinations possess magical qualities for inducing weight loss.

Crash diet formulas include grapefruit and coffee for days on end; celery and virtually nothing else; cottage cheese and little more. There are high-protein diets, "eat fat" diets, low-carbohydrate diets, all of which turn up under a variety of catchy names.

Such diets, obviously not well rounded, not providing all essential nutrients, have considerable potential for upsetting the body, for aggravating any previous small metabolic imbalances or even triggering some previously nonexisting ones. That they can drain vitality and produce fatigue should hardly come as a surprise.

Liquid reducing formulas are offered, with claims that they contain all required nutrients. Yet, as Drs. E. Cheraskin and W. M. Ringsdorf, Jr., of the University of Alabama have pointed out, "The fact is, no one has yet gathered the information necessary to compound such a formula. Any number of factors have yet to be isolated and identified. For example, there are antifatigue nutrients, found only in liver and wheat germ oil, so effective that adding either of these food items to the diet of animals who are strenuously exercised prolongs their endurance 300 or more percent. The wheat germ oil nutrient was only recently identified as a vegetable wax called octacosanol. There is also a nutrient factor in carrots that reduces the body's need for oxygen. No one knows what it is or how to refine it. Any one of the many unknown factors may be the very one you need the most. A liquid-diet formula is the last place you'll find it."

Fatigue and disease

Fatigue is associated with a very considerable variety of diseases.

Fatigue accompanied by fever can stem from atypical pneumonia, pulmonary tuberculosis, lung abscess, rheumatic fever, rheumatic heart disease, influenza, and infectious mononucleosis.

Fatigue with headache may occur in high blood pressure, hepatitis, polycythemia (a blood disorder), infectious mononucleosis, and in menopause.

Extreme fatigue may occur in histoplasmosis, a systemic fungal disease, which produces other symptoms such as emaciation, black stools, vomiting, diarrhea, and ulcerations on nose, ears, and pharynx.

Bronchiectasis, a chronic dilation of the air passages, which may occur as a complication of chronic sinus infection or asthma, or as an aftereffect of lung abscess, pneumonia, or tuberculosis, can produce marked fatigue along with shortness of breath and periodic coughing and the bringing up of foul-smelling phlegm.

Fatigue also may accompany malignancies such as leukemia (which also may produce joint pains, pallor, and bleeding of gums, nose, and skin) and stomach cancer (with other symptoms such as abdominal distention, heartburn, rapid satiation at meals, weight loss, vomiting of blood, and black, tarry stools).

Fatigue and deficiency states

As we've already noted, fad diets, which can lead to deficiencies of various essential nutrients, can cause fatigue for that very reason.

In addition to deficiency of folic acid, deficiencies of some other vitamins are well known for producing fatigue.

A deficiency of vitamin C may lead to fatigue along with other symptoms that may include lethargy, bleeding gums, loose teeth, and fragile bones.

A deficiency of vitamin B_1 may be accompanied by abnormal fatigue along with one or more other symptoms such as appetite and weight loss, numbness of hands and feet, leg cramps, emotional instability, difficulty in breathing and walking, rapid heartbeat, and fluid swelling of tissues.

Other causes

Some glandular disorders, notably hypothyroidism and adrenal insufficiency, or Addison's disease, may produce abnormal fatigue as one symptom. (See Chapter 8.)

Anemia can be a cause (Chapter 7).

Sleep disturbances, including some not always obvious to the victims, can account for seemingly psychogenic fatigue (Chapter 9).

Some medications may produce fatigue as a side effect, among them, anticonvulsants used for seizures, antianginals for angina pectoris, antiarrhythmic agents for heartbeat disturbances, anti-Parkinsonism agents, sulfonamides for infections, and oral contraceptives. (See Chapter 17.)

And hypoglycemia, or low blood sugar (Chapter 12), and cerebral allergy (Chapter 11) may sometimes account for abnormal fatigue, as may caffeinism (Chapter 6).

6. *The Caffeinism Connection*

It was Dr. John F. Greden, then of Walter Reed Army Medical Center and now associate professor of psychiatry at the University of Michigan, who brought the problem to light at a 1974 American Psychiatric Association meeting, along with some dramatic cases of people who benefited when the problem was recognized.

One, a young nurse married to an Army physician, sought help because of several weeks of light-headedness, tremulousness, breathlessness, headache, and irregular heartbeat. When examination disclosed nothing physically wrong, she was referred to a psychiatric outpatient clinic with a diagnosis of anxiety reaction attributed to worry that her husband would be sent to Vietnam.

But the young nurse refused to accept the diagnosis and, in fact, was the first to suspect the possible cause, and in about ten days managed to link her symptoms to coffee consumption. She had started making coffee by a different method that she found superior and so had been drinking ten to twelve cups a day. Her symptoms disappeared within thirty-six hours after she stopped drinking coffee. She was later challenged with caffeine twice, and each time the symptoms returned, only to disappear when the caffeine was eliminated.

Another case involved a 37-year-old military officer referred for psychiatric help after a two-year history of chronic anxiety. His symptoms occurred almost daily and included dizziness, tremulousness, apprehension about job performance, restlessness, frequent diarrhea, and persistent sleep problems. Three complete medical examinations turned up no explanation. Tranquilizers had little effect.

Finally, it was discovered that he drank eight to fourteen cups of coffee a day and often drank hot cocoa at bedtime. He liked only cola soft drinks and drank three or four a day. He was incredulous at the idea that caffeinism might be causing his problem, was unwilling at first to cut down on coffee, cocoa, and colas, but finally gave in. A few weeks later, he reported marked improvement.

The finding by Greden that large amounts of caffeine, taken in coffee and other beverages, including tea and cola drinks, and, in addition, in caffeine-containing medications, including some headache tablets, can produce symptoms mimicking those of chronic anxiety was soon to be confirmed by other investigators.

And, more recently, in another study, Greden has found indications that caffeinism may be a factor in some who suffer from depression and abnormal fatigue.

Caffeine: friend and/or foe

Americans are not quite up with Voltaire, a king of coffee drinkers, who is reputed to have consumed more than fifty cups a day. But we do drink up to half of world production, averaging about sixteen pounds per person per year.

According to legend, coffee was discovered a thousand or so years ago by Arabian shepherds who noticed their flocks gamboling about all night after eating the berries of the coffee plant and became impressed with coffee's stimulant qualities.

Those qualities, of course, are due to an ingredient, caffeine, which has a potent stimulating effect on the central nervous system.

Many, if not most, people have found numerous values in caffeine consumed in coffee and other beverages. It lessens, or at least masks, fatigue and relieves drowsiness, increases alertness, and may produce mild euphoria.

Drug makers have found many uses for it. It's the active ingredient in over-the-counter preparations to help people stay awake (the dose in a stimulant tablet is about the same, 100 milligrams, as the amount in a cup of coffee). It's commonly used in cold preparations to counter the drowsiness produced by antihistamine drugs. Because it constricts brain blood vessels, it's included in many prescription and over-the-counter drugs for headaches.

For a time, a dark cloud hung over coffee—or, more precisely, the caffeine in it—in terms of heart attacks. In 1963 came one of the first reports indicating a possible positive association between coffee and coronary heart disease. And in 1972 and 1973 other reports suggested that people who drink more than five cups a day have about twice as great a risk of having a heart attack as nondrinkers.

But then, more recently, came contradictory studies.

To be sure, caffeine can accelerate the heart rate, raise blood pressure, interfere with sleep, and elevate blood levels of fatty acids. But however impressive such circumstantial evidence might seem, is it enough to incriminate caffeine as a risk factor in coronary heart disease? The later studies provide some reassurance that it is not.

One was based on an analysis of multiphasic health checkup questionnaires completed by 197 men aged 40 to 79 years some time before they suddenly died. Comparison with data on other men comparable in age and other characteristics culled from 250,000 computerized multiphasic health checkup questionnaires showed no significant increase in the incidence of sudden deaths from heart attacks among those who drank coffee even in excess of six cups a day.

The other report came from the Framingham study, begun in 1949, one of the most intensive investigations into heart disease ever conducted. Records of daily coffee consumptions were kept for a twelve-year period in this continuing study that involves thousands of men and women in the Massachusetts community. No significant differences were found between coffee drinkers and noncoffee drinkers with regard to onset of coronary heart disease or the development of such heart disease manifestations as chest pain (angina pectoris) or heart attacks. The researchers also reported finding no significant relationship between coffee consumption and development of stroke and other heart and blood vessel problems not related to coronary heart disease.

But if the case against caffeine as a factor in heart disease is no longer all black, what of its relationship to other problems?

Ulcers? Caffeine does tend to stimulate stomach acid secretion. The stimulation appears to be mild and transitory in healthy people but may be sustained in those with ulcers, suggesting that people disposed to ulcers may be more sensitive and could do with moderation.

Heartburn? In some people, caffeine may contribute to heartburn. The mechanism seems to be twofold. Even as caffeine stimulates stomach acid secretion, it produces a slight decrease in the grip of the sphincter, or circular muscle, in the esophagus near the entrance to the stomach, and the decrease may be enough to allow some of the acid secretion to flow back out of the stomach and into the esophagus, producing heartburn.

The anxiety dose

Individual sensitivity varies, but for some people, Greden's original study indicated, as little as 250 milligrams of caffeine a day may be enough to produce symptoms mimicking those of chronic anxiety, among them, restlessness, irritability, muscle twitching, headache, insomnia, racing pulse, flushing, lethargy, nausea, vomiting, diarrhea, and chest pain.

If 250 milligrams seems like a large amount, many people exceed that intake almost daily. For example, three cups of coffee, two caffeine-containing headache tablets, and a caffeine-containing cola drink may be consumed in a morning, providing about 500 milligrams of caffeine.

In all surveys conducted among general populations, and among such subgroups as housewives and medical students, 20 to 30 percent of the respondents have been found to consume more than 500 to 600 milligrams of caffeine per day.

(An average cup of brewed coffee contains 100 to 150 milligrams of caffeine; instant coffee, 86 to 99 mg; decaffeinated coffee, 2 to 4 mg; tea, 60 to 75 mg; cocoa, 50 mg; cola drinks, 40 to 72 mg per 12 ounces; an ounce of milk chocolate, 3 mg, and of bittersweet chocolate, 25 mg. The caffeine content per tablet in such over-the-counter drugs as APC's, Anacin, Bromo Seltzer, Cope, Vanquish, Empirin compound, Midol, and Easy-Mens is about 32 mg; Excedrin, 60 mg; Pre-Mens, 66 mg; many cold preparations, 30 mg; many stimulants such as NoDoz, 100 mg. Among prescription drugs, Cafergot contains 100 mg per tablet; Darvon compound, 32 mg; Fiorinal, 40 mg; and Migral, 50 mg.)

Within a short time after Greden's original report that caffeinism could be misdiagnosed as an anxiety syndrome, several other investigators were confirming the finding. There followed a study in which a group of 135 psychiatric patients were checked during hospitalization and 25 percent were found to be "high" coffee drinkers, consuming more than five cups per day. The heaviest users scored significantly higher than others on an anxiety index and significantly more of them were diagnosed as "psychotic."

Depression and fatigue

Late in 1976, Dr. Greden and a group of associates carried out a study that took the caffeinism story a significant step further.

They administered a twenty-six-page questionnaire to eighty-three psychiatric inpatients sequentially hospitalized at the University of Michigan Medical Center and the

Ann Arbor Veterans Administration Hospital. The questionnaire covered types and amounts of caffeine consumed, self-observed effects of caffeine use, history of anxiety symptoms and other psychiatric problems. Then the researchers gave the patients tests for anxiety and depression.

Based on caffeine intake computations, the patients were divided into three groups: "low" consumers, who took in less than 250 milligrams a day; "moderate" consumers, with total intake of 250 to 749 milligrams a day; and "high" consumers, whose total intake exceeded 750 milligrams.

Even with the arbitrarily high level of 750 milligrams or greater set for high consumers—a lower level of 500 or 600 milligrams a day could have been chosen—22 percent of the patients fell into that category. Forty-two percent were moderate consumers and 36 percent low consumers.

Differences among the groups were notable. Sixty-one percent of the high consumers reported they often or almost always "tire quickly." This compared to 54 percent of moderate and only 24 percent of low consumers.

Significantly more of the highest consumers also reported getting in a state of tension over personal concerns, feeling that difficulties were piling up, feeling like crying, and feeling blue. Inversely, a much smaller percentage of the high consumers reported feeling pleasant, rested, happy, or content.

As caffeine intake increased, symptoms of anxiety increased and feelings of calmness decreased. A much larger percentage of high consumers reported frequent use of tranquilizers such as Valium, Librium, and Miltown and of sedatives.

One-half of the heavy consumers rated very high on a standard depression scale, suggesting severe depression.

Looking into sources of caffeine intake, the investigators found that the average high consumer got 75 percent from coffee, 10 to 15 percent from tea, 5 to 10 percent from cola drinks, and 5 to 10 percent from medications. Caffeine intake usually started by age 15 for the highest consumers and somewhat later for others, suggesting it may take years for the caffeinism syndrome to develop. One individual consumed an average of 400 milligrams a day via NoDoz tablets. Another's intake was a startling 4,000 milligrams a day, and, incredulous about this, the investigators took pains to substantiate the finding.

Despite their symptoms, few of the heavy consumers associated their problems with caffeine. In fact, some claimed that coffee or tea made them less depressed.

Greden and his associates were not surprised to find a high incidence of anxiety symptoms among high caffeine consumers. That could be expected from the pharmacology of the drug, its effects in the body. Not only is it a central nervous system stimulant; it also increases the body's output of norepinephrine, a hormone, which in excess is known to contribute to anxiety.

It's likely that some individuals are more sensitive than others to caffeine's effects. Whether a high percentage of such sensitive people is to be found among psychiatric patients is unknown as yet. But support for this possibility comes from a recent study by another investigator of unemployed auto workers which showed that when they consumed coffee under the stressful condition of having lost their jobs, their increase in norepinephrine output was greater than when they consumed it at nonstressful times and greater than that of control subjects.

Psychiatric patients have their own stresses, Greden points out, and it is possible that heavy caffeine intake at stressful times could help to provoke their symptoms.

Greden and his colleagues were most surprised by the high incidence of depression among the heavy consumers. One possible explanation is that some people may first become depressed and then "self-medicate" with caffeine. But it is also possible that chronic caffeine ingestion helps trigger depressive symptoms in certain people, and there are technical biological mechanisms already known by which the drug might do so.

In presenting the results of the study at the 1977 American Psychiatric Association annual meeting, Greden noted that its message for psychiatrists and other physicians is "that caffeinism probably can be found among a fairly large percentage of patients with psychiatric symptoms. Such subjects will only be identified, however, by history taking. Without inquiry, there will be no diagnosis; without diagnosis, there will be no relief."

It might be well, he suggests, for physicians treating patients with psychiatric disturbances and high caffeine intake to cut down their intake for a week or so and see what happens.

That's something, of course, that victims of anxiety, depression, or fatigue might want to try for themselves.

7. The Anemia Connection

Among major health problems afflicting Americans, none may be more misunderstood, neglected, and mistreated than anemia.

Anemia! Everybody knows, or thinks he knows, about it—just a matter of pale looks and under-par feelings to be quickly fixed with iron or vitamin tablets.

But when, not long ago, three people—a college girl, a mother of two, and a 34-year-old businessman—became anemic, all with the same symptoms, iron or vitamin tablets didn't help—and couldn't help. The girl's anemia came from a thyroid disorder, the woman's from a previously unsuspected bleeding ulcer, and the man's from a medication that, although usually valuable, was affecting his whole blood supply, and if that hadn't been discovered in time and stopped, he could have lost his life.

These cases suggest one aspect of anemia: that it has many causes. Another is that it can wear many guises.

When very mild, anemia can produce a vague sense of easy fatigability or lack of energy. When not so mild, you are likely to be well aware of the fatigability and reduced energy level and there may also be irritability and vague abdominal pains. When severe, anemia can lead to exhaustion and apathy, and any or many of a wide range of symptoms, including appetite loss, nausea, vomiting, diarrhea; skin with yellowish tint; tongue soreness; crawling, prickling sensations of hands and feet; shortness of breath; palpitations; pounding headaches; spots before the eyes; and clouding of the mind or even psychotic behavior.

Common and mismanaged

More than a dozen years ago, it became clear that anemia was far more prevalent than had been supposed. There were reports then of the discovery of anemia in at least 20 percent of all patients admitted to general hospitals, no matter for what reason.

The medical reports were indicating then that although the total incidence was unknown, mild anemia might affect many, and moderate or severe anemia was very common in certain groups, such as young children, the elderly, and pregnant women.

There was medical concern, then, over a common public misconception that the surest way to re-energize "tired blood" was to take a vitamin-mineral mixture; much precious time was being wasted through such often fruitless therapy.

There was also concern over the failings of many physicians to treat anemia properly, physicians who, as one distinguished hematologist put it, "believe one might as well give any patient who has anemia vitamins and iron, cobalt and copper, intrinsic factor and liver, desiccated stomach and a few other things and expect all will go well." Using such a shotgun approach, they made little or no effort to find out what was causing the anemia.

At the time, an editorial in the *Journal of the American Medical Association* cautioned: "Anemia is the signal for a careful diagnosis, not for an expensive capsule that is likely only to delay diagnosis."

Has the situation changed? Today, anemia remains common. If anything, it may be even more common. Among new influences to make it more common is the widespread use of oral contraceptives. Another spotlighted not long ago: the taking of blood for diagnostic tests. In a study at a major New York hospital, 40 percent of a group of patients who were not anemic when they entered the hospital were found to be anemic before they were ready to be discharged, and the reason turned out to be the withdrawal of blood for tests. The study indicated that unless there was careful planning to eliminate unnecessary tests and reduce the amount of blood required, "blood test anemia" could become a significant problem.

Is the treatment of anemia better now than a dozen or so years ago? It can be. It often is. But too often it isn't.

Not only is much of the public still confused and uninformed about anemia; it appears that many physicians are too. They still use the old shotgun approach. They still seem to forget that anemia is a signal and its cause has to be ferreted out and treated if the patient is to be cured. "They have developed," worries one well-known hematologist, "a sort of reflex and reach for iron, vitamin B_{12}, folic acid, or some other readily available therapeutic agent instead of trying to identify exactly what is wrong."

It is easily possible for some people with emotional and behavioral disturbances and/or other seemingly psychosomatic physical symptoms to be victims of anemia—either unknowing victims, or uselessly self-treated, or even medically mismanaged.

The blood picture

Anemia means an abnormal condition of the blood, and it is best understood with some awareness of the workings of that rather remarkable internal sea.

Flowing through some sixty thousand miles of arteries, veins and capillaries to constantly bathe all parts of the body, blood is rich in many materials, including red and white blood cells.

The white are protective. Prick your finger, for example, and if bacteria enter and begin to multiply, white cells are mobilized at the site to fend them off.

But day in and day out, it's the red cells that maintain life. They are saucer-shaped particles so tiny it requires three thousand to cover the space of an inch, and there are enough of them in the blood—about thirty trillion—to encircle the earth four times if lined up in a beadlike chain.

Red cells owe their color to hemoglobin, a pigment with great affinity for and ability to hold on to oxygen. And it is through hemoglobin that red cells carry life-supporting oxygen from the lungs to all body tissues.

Created largely in the marrow of short, flat bones, red cells can function for up to 120 days and then, worn out, are removed from the circulation and destroyed in the spleen.

Protein and iron from foods go into the making of hemoglobin. Other dietary substances, including vitamins and minerals, help build the red cells.

And if all goes well, red cell and hemoglobin formation keeps up with body requirements. Each hour, some ten billion new hemoglobin-filled red cells are needed to replace those worn out.

Anemia develops when red cells are inadequate in number or in the amount of hemoglobin they contain.

Iron deficiency anemia

Iron deficiency anemia is the most common type of anemia. Too little iron leads to underproduction of hemoglobin and oxygen deficiency for body tissues. The symptoms may include weakness, easy fatigability, and irritability. There may be skin pallor, heartburn, flatulence, vague abdominal pains, and a capricious appetite suggesting neurosis. Iron deficiency anemia also has been linked to such bizarre behavior as the eating of dirt or clay by pregnant women, the eating of trays of ice cubes by adults, and the chewing on plaster and paint chips, with risk of lead poisoning, by children.

Total body iron amounts to only about 5 or 6 grams, roughly a fifth of an ounce. Each day in a healthy person experiencing no abnormal bleeding about 1 milligram is lost in urine, sweat, and cast-off cells. The loss must be made up by diet, and a good diet contains about 6 milligrams of iron per 1,000 calories. Not all of this is absorbed; in fact, recent studies show that on an average only about 5 to 10 percent is utilized; the rest is excreted.

Thus, if a good average diet provides 6 milligrams per 1,000 calories, or a total of 12 to 18 milligrams of iron per day, the absorption rate of 5 to 10 percent would give the body just about enough new iron to counter the normal loss of the old.

But recent surveys indicate that 20 percent of U.S. women of childbearing age have iron deficiency anemia, and adolescent girls on the average are getting 30 percent less iron than they need. Fewer men are affected but men are not immune.

Through all the years of menstruation, most women are in precarious iron balance. The average woman may take in less iron than a man because she may eat less in total or less of iron-rich foods in particular. (Meats are good iron sources, providing 2 to 3 milligrams in a three-ounce serving, with liver in particular providing several times that much; an egg contains 1 milligram; oysters, sardines, and shrimp provide 2½ to 5 milligrams per three-ounce serving; most green vegetables provide 1 to 4 milligrams per cup; and other good sources include dry beans, nuts, prunes, dates, and raisins, each containing about 5 milligrams per cup.)

And women lose much more iron than healthy men. Normally, as much as 28 milligrams may be lost in menstrual blood. On an iron-poor diet, iron deficiency may occur even with normal menstrual loss. Increased menstrual flow adds to the risk.

And investigators have found that women are often unaware that they are losing more than the normal amount of menstrual blood, even several times more than normal, because menstrual pads absorb blood so efficiently that false impressions are obtained.

Normal menstrual volume is in the range of 35 to 70 cubic centimeters, or 1/15 to 2/15 of a pint. Yet, as examples of how excess volume may be overlooked, one investigator tells of two intelligent, medically trained women with anemia whose extracted pads were found to contain an excess of 200 cubic centimeters per period and neither one had been aware that her blood loss was unusual.

Iron "steals"

Almost paradoxically, Harvard investigators not long ago found that iron deficiency may even cause excessive menstrual bleeding. This is because hemoglobin has great affinity for whatever iron is available in the body, and when there is a shortage of iron, hemoglobin may steal iron from an enzyme involved in muscle function. The result can be weakness of uterine muscular elements that leads to inadequate contraction of tiny uterine blood vessels and continued heavy flow. In patients with heavy flow problems, the Harvard physicians have found that increased iron intake may produce marked improvement.

Recently, too, University of Chicago investigators have reported that a similar steal mechanism may explain the otherwise mysterious symptoms of chronic fatigue, nervousness, dizziness, and headaches in some women *who do not have measurable anemia*. With iron stores depleted, iron may be diverted from tissue enzymes to hemoglobin, and some women with adequate red cell hemoglobin may have "tired tissues" rather than "tired blood."

Other causes

Every case of iron deficiency anemia deserves careful checking out. Not only is it risky to assume that because certain symptoms are present the problem is anemia and then to take readily available iron-containing preparations; it is also risky—"sinful," one hematologist puts it—for a physician, after establishing by simple blood test that the anemia is an iron deficiency type, to simply prescribe iron.

The deficiency may or may not be due to inadequate iron intake. It may, for example, be due to poor absorption, as in celiac disease, a digestive system disturbance in which ability to digest and utilize fats and some other food materials is impaired as the result of sensitivity to the gluten component of wheat and rye.

When full-blown, celiac disease produces flatulence and large, foul-smelling, frothy stools containing much fat. The abdomen may be swollen and there may be recurrent attacks of diarrhea alternating with constipation. But recent reports indicate that perhaps one-third of patients—adults and children—with celiac disease are going undiagnosed because they do not have the typical complex of symptoms. Some simply have iron deficiency anemia. Celiac disease, and the iron deficiency accompanying it, can be overcome by treatment that may include for a time a diet free from gluten and fat.

More often, what needs to be considered in iron deficiency anemia is abnormal bleeding. In a woman, it may be important to check on the possibility of excessive menstruation. And especially in men and postmenopausal women, a common source of blood loss is gastrointestinal bleeding. It doesn't have to be massive bleeding. A loss of a few cubic centimeters daily over an extended period can result in iron deficiency.

Such loss can be caused by hemorrhoids, by ulcers, by diverticular disease. In diverticular disease, there may be hundreds of abnormal little outpouchings of the colon, or large bowel, that may become inflamed and may bleed. Diverticular disease is a common problem and a remediable one, sometimes with the aid of a high-fiber, bulk-producing diet.

Sometimes, hiatus hernia may account for blood loss. It's a condition, also called diaphragmatic hernia, in which the stomach protrudes abnormally upward through the diaphragm. Hiatus hernia is common and commonly produces no symptoms and requires no treatment. But sometimes it may allow stomach contents to move back upward into the esophagus, producing heartburn and pain under the chest and, in some cases, bleeding.

In some people, chronic use of aspirin may cause gastrointestinal bleeding, enough to produce iron deficiency anemia.

And malignancies of the intestinal tract can also produce blood loss.

Proper treatment

Whenever iron deficiency anemia is diagnosed, the possibility of blood loss should be considered. It may be possible for the physician to eliminate some potential causes of loss on the basis of physical examination and the patient's history. To check on others may require X-ray and other studies of the gastrointestinal tract.

Even as the physician checks for the source of bleeding, he can use iron therapy, which usually does not interfere with the search and can make the patient feel better.

A simple iron preparation, such as ferrous sulfate, can be used. Too often, experts say, physicians stop iron treatment too soon, or patients do. Although an iron supplement may correct the anemia within a month or so, three to six months of treatment may be needed to build up iron stores in patients who have had a significant degree of anemia.

Folic acid deficiency anemia

While still outranked by iron deficiency, folic acid deficiency has become an increasingly common cause of anemia.

Folic acid is an essential B vitamin present in many natural foods—leafy vegetables, meat and fish, and dairy foods. Unfortunately, it's rapidly destroyed by heat. A deficiency can occur when foods containing the vitamin are lacking in the diet or are cooked too long.

The body may also be starved of folic acid by contraceptive pills which, in some women, interfere seriously with its absorption from food. The same effect may be produced in some cases by various drugs, antimalarials, anticonvulsants used for epilepsy, methotrexate, which is sometimes used for severe psoriasis, and alcohol (heavy drinkers are prone to folic acid deficiency).

World Health Organization studies show folic acid deficiency in one-third to one-half of all pregnant women throughout the world, including the United States. This is because the fetus makes inroads into maternal folic acid stores.

A deficiency of folic acid can interfere with production of blood cells. Typically, with the deficiency, the red cells are abnormally large and abnormally shaped, and they have an abnormally short life-span. Much activity goes on in the bone marrow where red cells are produced, but many of the deficient cells are destroyed even before they begin to circulate in the blood.

Depending upon the degree of folic acid deficiency, anemia may be mild, moderate, or severe. Onset of symptoms may be insidious. At some point, weakness and easy fatigability may become apparent. Irritability, too, may be noted. And in some cases the symptoms may include sleeplessness and forgetfulness. Folic acid deficiency also can make the tongue sore, red, swollen, smooth, and glistening.

When suspected, folic acid deficiency is readily diagnosed through a simple test to measure the level of folic acid in a sample of blood. The deficiency—and the anemia and other changes accompanying it—responds dramatically in most cases to treatment with an oral dose of just 1 milligram of folic acid a day. Larger doses are not needed and are wasteful.

B_6 and sideroblastic anemia

Affecting mostly men, producing symptoms like those of any severe anemia, sideroblastic anemia is a mysterious anemia.

The red blood cells look much like those of iron deficiency anemia—pale and small. But there is no shortage of iron; in fact, iron concentration in the blood is increased.

The trouble is that the iron is not being incorporated into hemoglobin, and the red cells, lacking hemoglobin, are pale and small and unable to properly transport oxygen.

The anemia is related to pyridoxine (vitamin B_6).

A relative newcomer among vitamins, B_6 was first identified in 1934 when it cured a skin disorder in rats. Not until 1952 was there any evidence that it is essential in man.

Now it's known to be needed for proper body handling of proteins and carbohydrates and to have a key role in the production of hemoglobin. In the early stages of hemoglobin synthesis, B_6 enters into a critical chemical reaction, and if the vitamin is not there, the reaction cannot proceed and hemoglobin production stops, resulting in anemia.

Not much of the vitamin is needed, although exact requirements are still in question. The vitamin is widely distributed in foods. But when vegetables are frozen they may lose 25 percent of their B_6 content; the high sterilization temperatures in canning destroy the vitamin; and in the milling of cereal grains to produce refined white flour, much of the vitamin may be lost.

Certain drugs, notably isoniazid and cycloserine, which are useful in treating tuberculosis, induce anemia, apparently by interfering with B_6 activity. The anemia can be corrected by giving the vitamin.

But some people, mostly men, otherwise healthy, develop anemia as the result of a special need for large amounts of B_6. A hereditary pattern has been demonstrated in some families.

Fortunately, when the anemia is identified correctly, as it can be readily by blood and bone marrow tests, it responds to 50 to 200 milligrams of B_6 by mouth a day. The excess iron floating in the blood disappears, going into hemoglobin; the hemoglobin is incorporated into normal red cells; the whole blood picture becomes normal; and the anemia is eliminated.

Not-always-obvious pernicious anemia

There were almost two dozen patients admitted to a large hospital in upstate New York. A few sought help directly from the hospital, but most were referred by their personal physicians. It was to turn out that all had the same problem but not exactly the same symptoms. In not one case was the right diagnosis made before admission to the hospital.

Many of the patients had complained of weakness, breathing difficulty, weight and appetite loss. Others suffered from one or more such symptoms as fatigability, memory impairment, abdominal discomfort, burning or tingling sensations, dizziness, vomiting, constipation, sore tongue, chest pain, cough, unsteadiness, abnormal gait, difficulty in walking.

All had pernicious anemia. Why hadn't that diagnosis been made by referring physicians, who in some cases had observed the patients over weeks or months?

For one thing, pernicious anemia has often been thought of as an anemia in which, invariably, tongue inflammation and abnormal sensations or numbness of the legs can be expected. But only three of the patients complained of a sore tongue, and only five had abnormal sensations or numbness of the legs.

For another thing, some physicians seem to be unaware that pernicious anemia is really a multisystem disease that not only affects the blood and leads to anemia but also affects other tissues and systems, including brain, nervous system, liver, and digestive system.

It's an insidious disease that occurs most often after the age of 50 but can strike younger people. Commonly, such general symptoms of anemia as weakness, shortness of breath, and palpitation do not occur until the disease has been present for some time. Often, the first indications may be mild tongue soreness and pins-and-needle sensations of hands or feet. Varying from one patient to another, gastrointestinal symptoms may appear earlier or later and may include nausea, vomiting, diarrhea, abdominal pain, and appetite and weight loss.

In almost half of all cases, nervous system symptoms develop and may include memory impairment, clouding of mental awareness, sometimes euphoria or feelings of exaggerated well-being, and in advanced cases even psychotic behavior may be triggered.

The cause of pernicious anemia is a deficiency of vitamin B_{12}, but not because of lack of the vitamin in the diet. An amount in the diet as small as 1 microgram a day is sufficient, and a microgram is a millionth of a gram, and a gram, in turn, is only one-thirtieth of an ounce—astonishing in view of the fact that B_{12} is essential for the formation of red blood cells, normal growth, and maintenance of health of nerve cells.

In pernicious anemia, absorption of B_{12} is impaired for lack of adequate amounts of a material, intrinsic factor, which is a normal constituent of the gastric juice.

Many tests are available to diagnose pernicious anemia. One of the most useful is the Schilling test, in which a small amount of radioactive vitamin B_{12} is administered by mouth and the amount of the material excreted in the urine is measured. The test shows whether the vitamin is being properly absorbed.

Treatment is directed at overcoming the vitamin deficiency and at creating and maintaining an adequate body reserve of the vitamin. These goals can be achieved by injections of 50 to 100 micrograms of the vitamin every one to seven days for two to four months, followed by maintenance injections about once a month. The injections, of course, bypass the gastrointestinal tract and eliminate the need for intrinsic factor to permit absorption.

Hypothyroid anemia

The college girl mentioned earlier in this chapter, whose anemia was the result of thyroid disorder, is no rare case. Nor is an older man whose anemia was treated first with iron and, when that did no good, with vitamin B_{12}, which was equally useless.

In addition to the usual symptoms of anemia, he had dry skin and unusual sensitivity to cold temperatures. Because these could be indications of hypothyroidism, or underfunctioning of the thyroid gland, he was tested for thyroid activity. According to the first test, nothing was wrong with the gland. Fortunately, a repeat test was done and this time showed hypothyroidism. When he was treated with thyroid extract to make up for the gland's underfunctioning, all his symptoms, including those of anemia, responded, although it took several months before he was entirely free of them.

Exactly how thyroid deficiency (see also Chapter 8) causes anemia is not clear. Thyroid hormone secretions are important in the functioning of every organ, tissue, and body cell. With deficiency, there may be interference with absorption and use of vitamins such as B_{12}. Consumption of oxygen by the tissues may be reduced and this may play a role in anemia. Thyroid deficiency also can be responsible in some women for excessive menstruation, which in turn may contribute to the development of anemia.

The difficulty with thyroid deficiency is not in treatment. Thyroid medication is effective. But tests used to detect thyroid deficiency, while reliable when deficiency is severe, are sometimes inaccurate in mild to moderate hypothyroidism. Many physicians, experienced in diagnosis and treatment of thyroid problems, are aware of the possibility of error with tests, and if they are suspicious, based on a patient's symptoms, that gland functioning may be under par, they will repeat a test. Others, however, may dismiss the possibility of hypothyroidism after one negative test.

G6PD and an anemia of men

G6PD deficiency is one of the most common genetic abnormalities of man, occurring throughout southern Europe, the Middle East, Africa, and the Orient, with a significant incidence in blacks, Sephardic Jews, Greeks, Arabs, and East Indians. In the United States, it occurs in about 12 percent of black males and in 2 to 20 percent of males of Mediterranean ancestry, depending on geographic origin.

It is totally innocuous, producing no symptoms, causing no difficulties at all except under certain conditions involving use of some drugs or the presence of severe infection. Then it leads to the destruction of many red blood cells and thus anemia, with the usual symptoms.

The abnormality is a deficiency of an enzyme, G6PD (glucose-6-phosphate dehydrogenase), normally present in red cells. The deficiency is determined by a sex-linked gene, affecting only men.

Particular attention was called to G6PD some years ago when a mysterious anemia developed in some members of the armed forces who were being treated with drugs to overcome or prevent malaria. The missing enzyme proved to be the reason.

Now it's known that in the presence of the enzyme deficiency, anemia may be produced by other drugs as well, including aspirin, sulfa compounds, phenacetin (an ingredient in some headache remedies), and nitrofurantoin, an antibacterial drug sometimes used in treating urinary tract infections.

A test for the deficiency can be done in any physician's office, allowing anyone who has it to avoid use of drugs that may bring on an episode of red cell destruction and anemia.

A potentially fatal anemia

Aplastic anemia is a form of anemia in which there is partial or complete shutdown of bone marrow production of blood cells.

Sometimes it can be of unknown cause. But there are a number of known causes. Aplastic anemia may sometimes follow as a complication of viral hepatitis or of the use of anticancer drugs or of radiation to combat malignancy. It may be triggered by a chemical such as benzene or arsenic.

Occasionally, it may stem from use of ordinarily valuable drugs, among them, sulfa compounds and the antibiotic chloramphenicol employed for infections, gold compounds and phenylbutazone for arthritic conditions, and the antimalarial drug quinacrine.

Usually, aplastic anemia develops in insidious fashion. Even when the cause is a chemical or a drug, weeks and sometimes months may elapse before symptoms appear. When symptoms do appear, the general symptoms of anemia, including fatigue and weakness, are usually severe. The skin and mucous membranes develop a waxy pallor and black-and-blue spots may appear. Sometimes there is bleeding from nose and mouth.

Aplastic anemia can be diagnosed by blood studies and by the appearance of bone marrow in a sample taken by puncture of the breastbone.

When the cause is a toxic chemical or a drug, spontaneous recovery often occurs when the agent is removed. In cases of unknown cause, blood transfusions and various other measures may be required.

Early diagnosis is essential. Self-treatment, or shotgun treatment by a physician, could be deadly.

Getting the right help

If you suspect, because of fatigability, weakness, pallor, or any other symptom, that you may be anemic, see a physician. Don't try self-treatment.

When you see a physician, you have a right to expect him to do blood tests to determine whether anemia is actually present. Indications of anemia include reduction in hemoglobin or red cell count.

If anemia is present, you have a right to expect the physician to try to determine the cause, and you should be suspicious if he doesn't do so. You should expect him to take a thorough history of all your symptoms, of any medications you are taking, of family background and family medical history. Depending upon individual circumstances, there may be need for further testing, possibly bone marrow and other studies.

You have a right to have the physician tell you the type of anemia you have, the suspected cause, why the suspicion, what if any other possible causes there might be, and the plan of treatment.

In short, you should get from the physician more than "Just a bit of anemia. Take this." If you don't, go elsewhere.

And if you do get more but don't get results—clear-cut improvement—within three months, you have the right, and the necessity, to ask for a consultation with a blood specialist (hematologist).

8. *A Diversity of Emotional/Behavioral Disturbances and Errant Glands*

When, some years ago, Dr. Martha Schon of the Neuropsychiatric Service at Memorial Hospital in New York City did a thorough evaluation of two dozen patients with untreated thyroid gland deficiency, she found that they could be mistaken easily for neurotics.

They were easily fatigued, irritable, nervous, and emotionally explosive. Although they regretted their behavior, they were unable to control it. They suffered, too, from decreased sexual function, diffuse muscular pain, vision disturbances, and speech difficulties.

Once the thyroid deficiency was corrected, Dr. Schon found, most symptoms, emotional and physical, decreased or disappeared, to be replaced by a sense of well-being and a feeling of integration of personality.

Brain as well as body functioning is sensitive to the activities of endocrine gland hormones. And that psychiatric as well as physical symptoms can accompany malfunctioning of a gland has been known for many years.

Depending upon the gland involved and the degree of its malfunctioning, there may be mild, moderate, or severe personality changes, anxiety, depression, fatigue, apathy, intellectual impairment, or even psychosis.

Sometimes emotional/behavioral complaints are the first

manifestations; they can seem psychogenic. Sometimes the physical complaints may be vague and diffuse; they too may be dismissed as "all in the mind" unless there is a high index of suspicion.

The interplay

Until about a century ago, the single controlling force for complex body processes was considered to be the nervous system, of which the brain is part.

But there were puzzling, unanswered questions. It was difficult, for example, to explain the size differences of people, the body changes occurring at puberty, and the variations of vigor and energy in terms of the nervous system alone.

Another influence had to be at work and eventually it was found in the endocrine system. That system of glands differs markedly from other gland systems of the body.

The latter—sweat, salivary, and other exocrine glands—are glands of external secretion. They pour their products through ducts, or tubes, to sites where they have local purposes.

The endocrines—glands of internal secretion—have no ducts. Instead, they send their secretions into the bloodstream to be carried to, and exert effects at, sites far removed.

The endocrine glands are widely separated in the body and they differ markedly in appearance.

The pituitary is a round body, about the size of a large green pea, attached by a stalk to the hypothalamus. The butterfly-shaped thyroid is deep in the throat. The parathyroids, near to or attached to the thyroid, are four little bodies (two pairs) that resemble BB shots.

The adrenals arise like mushrooms, one atop each kidney. The pancreas, a large gland (about 6 inches long), lies against the back wall of the abdomen. It might appear, superficially, not to belong to the endocrine system since it has a duct leading into the intestine. But it also contains tiny segments called islets, which form an endocrine gland, pouring their secretions into the bloodstream.

The gonads, or sex glands, consist of testes in men and ovaries in women. And there are two other glands in the system: the pineal, in the upper part of the brain, about which as yet little is known; and the thymus, behind the breastbone, which appears to be involved in establishing the body's immunity, or defense, system.

The secretions of hormones sent by the endocrine glands through the bloodstream to various parts of the body act like messengers. The word "hormone" comes from a Greek word meaning *to excite* or *stir up*. And the hormonal secretions actually create no processes but instead give orders for certain processes to speed up or slow down.

The endocrine glands are interdependent. What happens to one affects the others. If one gland is removed or its functioning changes, the functioning of others is altered.

As one example of the interdependency, the pituitary secretes one hormone that serves to stimulate the adrenal glands. In turn, the adrenals secrete one hormone that travels to the pituitary and signals the latter to slow production of the adrenal-arousing pituitary hormone.

In fact, the pituitary secretes various hormones to stir up each of the other endocrine glands, each of which responds, as do the adrenals, with hormones to signal the pituitary when they've had enough stimulation.

Until recently, the pituitary was believed to be the body's "master gland," but it is now evident that it is no monarch on its own. It is connected to a brain area called the hypothalamus. And the hypothalamus produces secretions that affect pituitary functioning.

That the endocrine system and the autonomic nervous system, the branch of the nervous system that operates without conscious control and governs the activities of the heart muscle and muscles of the digestive and respiratory systems, work together closely is clear.

Consider, for example, what happens when, for any reason, you experience an alarm reaction. From the nervous system, a message comes to the adrenals, which then secrete a hormone that increases heart action and narrows blood vessels so blood is pushed through them with more force; the hormone also relaxes and enlarges the airways so more air can reach the lungs more quickly; in addition, the hormone reaches the pituitary, which responds to it by secreting hormones to cause the thyroid, parathyroids, and even the gonads to secrete hormones, all to complete the almost instantaneous mustering of the body and mind forces to deal with the stress situation, to fight or flee, and to account for some of the superhuman feats of action that are often exhibited under stress.

The relationship between endocrine and nervous systems is two-way. Nerve impulses influence glands and glands influence nerves. Emotions affect the autonomic nervous system, which in turn affects gland activity. And glands work through the nervous system and influence emotions.

Thyroid disturbances

The one-ounce thyroid gland was one of the first endocrine glands discovered. And there is an old medical saying that only a few grams of thyroid hormone can make the difference between an idiot and an Einstein.

The thyroid controls body metabolism, the rate at which chemical processes go on and energy is used. Minute thyroid secretions, something less than a spoonful a year, are responsible for much of body heat production. They help maintain the circulatory system; without them, the heartbeat slows, many blood vessels close down, and fluid leaks out of the bloodstream. They're necessary for muscle health; in their absence, muscles become sluggish and infiltrated with fat. They also heighten the sensitivity of nerves.

They play a vital role, from the beginning, in brain development. In infancy, absence of thyroid hormones results in cretinism. The symptoms include failure to thrive, torpid behavior, a hoarse cry. Within a year or two, mental growth retardation becomes apparent. With early recognition of the extreme thyroid deficiency, all of this can be avoided by thyroid hormone treatment.

Total lack of thyroid hormone is rare. But unbalanced thyroid functioning, so that thyroid secretions are either too much or too little, is not rare at all.

Many manifestations of severe malfunctioning are well known and almost unmistakable.

With severe hyperthyroidism, the gland producing grossly excessive amounts of hormone, the victim is nervous and irritable, tires easily, may lose weight to the point of emaciation despite good appetite. Often, the eyes protrude and the skin is warm and moist. In addition, the pulse may race, blood pressure may shoot up.

In the other direction, the severely hypothyroid individual, whose gland produces grossly inadequate amounts of secretions, experiences a slowing of the whole body economy. Weakness and listlessness develop; the skin becomes dry; there is heightened sensitivity to cold; memory is poor; sex drive is low; speech may become slow and thick.

Such effects are usually readily recognized for what they are by physicians and even by some patients. They are the classical symptoms of severe thyroid dysfunction, and people who have them are quickly given medical tests that can confirm diagnosis and allow effective treatment to be started.

In one test, for basal metabolism, the patient inhales oxygen and the amount left in the exhaled air shows how much the body has used and indicates how the thyroid is functioning. The test is little used today because of the problems involved in it: the patient must go without breakfast and spend considerable time lying motionless.

A variety of other thyroid function tests is available. In one, a capsule of radioactive iodine is swallowed and a counter device detects how much gets into the thyroid gland. In another, the amount of protein-bound iodine in the blood is measured and provides an indication of thyroid functioning. There are still others, including one that measures the output of a pituitary gland hormone that stimulates thyroid activity.

Once thyroid disturbance is diagnosed, treatment can be gratifyingly effective.

For hyperthyroidism, an antithyroid drug, such as propylthiouracil or methimazole, may be used to suppress excessive secretion. Over a period of some months, thyroid functioning may be brought down to a normal range and drug treatment can be stopped. This method of treatment may not be suitable for some people, including about 9 percent who develop fever, skin outbreaks, or other reactions because of drug sensitivity.

Alternatively, surgery or radioactive iodine treatment may be used. Surgery, called subtotal thyroidectomy, removes part of the thyroid gland, enough to eliminate the excess of secretions. Injection of radioactive iodine, in amounts many times those employed for testing thyroid function, also may bring thyroid activity down to normal.

For hypothyroidism, simple replacement therapy works. The patients regularly take thyroid hormone pills, either extracted from animal glands or made synthetically, in a dosage suitable for supplementing gland production.

Missed diagnoses

It is not unusual for thyroid disorders to go undetected and unsuspected for long periods or even to be missed entirely.

Delays in diagnosis may occur because the disorders may develop slowly, and if the first symptoms are limited to such vague ones as weakness, fatigue, nervousness, and irritability, they may be attributed by patients, and sometimes by physicians, to other causes.

Studies in recent years have produced findings on the many guises thyroid disturbance can assume.

For example, when a middle-aged woman was admitted to a Los Angeles hospital after a year of progressive weight loss, weakness, and episodes of diarrhea, she weighed only sixty-five pounds and was thought to have gastrointestinal cancer. But tests failed to disclose a malignancy. She continued to lose weight in the hospital. Finally, two weeks after admission, the possibility of thyroid disease was considered and was confirmed by tests. The diagnosis had been missed at first because she had none of the usual symptoms of severe hyperthyroidism. With drug treatment to control her excessive thyroid activity, she rapidly regained weight, strength, and health.

A 57-year-old man was admitted to the same hospital after his family, for a year, had found him increasingly unmanageable, subject to bouts of agitation, restlessness, and overactivity. Sometimes he became combative; sometimes he had delusions. After evaluation in the hospital, he was admitted to a psychiatric ward with a diagnosis of psychosis.

In the ward, he couldn't sit still, insisted on helping to wash windows, mop floors, bus trays. He rarely slept and was constantly asking for extra portions of food. After two weeks of this behavior, a doctor in the ward suspected thyroid disease. Tests showed severe thyroid overactivity. The patient was transferred to the medical division of the hospital and was treated with an antithyroid drug. He quickly calmed down and could be discharged in good health.

Although a sizable proportion of patients with severe hyperthyroidism may display erratic, even bizarre, behavior, the behavioral disturbances may be misinterpreted as being the results of psychiatric rather than physical illness.

In fact, as Dr. Gregory M. Brown, professor of psychiatry at the University of Toronto, has pointed out, "At one time it was thought that anxiety or stress was the cause of hyperthyroidism and there is a considerable body of literature on the relationship. If anxiety were in fact the cause, it would be on the basis of activation by the hypothalamus of the pituitary, which in turn would activate the thyroid gland, but that is not the usual sequence. In the vast majority of cases, plasma thyroid-stimulating hormone (TSH) levels are quite low, which means that the pituitary is not hypersecreting TSH and the brain is not being stimulated by anxiety to drive the thyroid. The anxiety seen in hyperthyroidism is probably the result rather than causal factor in thyroid hormone hypersecretion."

Investigators who have studied hyperthyroid patients have found serious mental disturbances in as many as 20 percent. But the disturbances are not uniform in nature. Anxiety and depression are frequent. So are destructive impulsivity on the one hand and social withdrawal on the other.

At the University of North Carolina, physicians studied ten hyperthyroid patients with mental disturbances. Four had increased difficulty in concentrating and impairment of recent memory. One had loss of both visual and hearing acuity. Many had difficulty with simple arithmetic. Fatigue, anxiety, and irritability were common complaints. Two patients complained of depression. Two suffered from delusions of being persecuted and one of the two had hallucinations in which she saw "swarms of bees" flying toward her. In all these cases, there was remarkable improvement following treatment for the thyroid dysfunction.

Other bizarre forms of hyperthyroidism have occasionally been reported: myasthenia, or muscle weakness; periodic paralysis of muscles; severe chest pain; ankle swelling; and comatose states.

Hardly any less than overfunctioning, underfunctioning of the thyroid can produce many deceptive mental as well as physical symptoms.

Hypothyroidism

Recognition of a state of low thyroid functioning dates back only about a century. Originally called myxedema, it was first appreciated in England.

And when, in 1888, a British commission, which had been appointed five years before to look into the strange condition, issued its report on a study of one hundred cases, it noted that all were slow in thought and response, suffered from poor memory, and almost half had delusions, hallucinations, or frank insanity.

More than a dozen years later, Dr. G. R. Murray, a British physician who was first to treat myxedema successfully, produced a treatise, *A System of Medicine,* in which he detailed how myxedema symptoms developed.

Often first to appear, he observed, was listlessness, so that ordinary daily tasks previously performed without much effort became irksome. Commonly, sensitivity to cold followed. Early in the disease there might sometimes be auditory or visual hallucinations. Murray also noted that all myxedema sufferers—myxedema, in fact, was severe hypothyroidism—were slow to comprehend a new subject or follow a new line of thought. Many were irritable. Unless treatment was started early, Murray pointed out, mania, melancholia, or dementia might develop.

About the turn of the century, physicians became aware of the relationship between thyroid deficiency and behavioral abnormalities through experience with some patients with huge goiters (thyroid gland enlargements). When the goiters became so large as to threaten to suffocate them by compressing the windpipe, the unfortunate patients underwent surgical removal of the thyroid as a last resort. This was at a time when thyroid replacement therapy was not available. And the surgery was, indeed, a last resort, the lesser of two evils, for with removal of the thyroid, severe behavioral as well as other changes followed.

In one case reported in the medical literature, a 10-year-old boy required thyroid gland removal. Six months later, a "marked psychical change," as it was called, was noted. Once a bright and lively youngster, the boy became quiet and retiring; growth stopped; his facial expression became that of an idiot, his hair spare, his speech slow. He could learn nothing in school and left at age 14. Unable to work, he also became incapable of thinking.

Goiter today is no longer as common as it once was. The cause of simple goiter is lack of adequate iodine in the soil and in drinking water. The thyroid gland is a factory producing its secretions for which iodine is an essential raw material. If iodine is lacking, hormone production slumps. When the slump is great enough, signals come to the thyroid from elsewhere urging an increase in hormone output. Trying to oblige, the gland may increase in size in a blind effort to increase its output, and the enlargement may produce a noticeable lump in the throat.

There are many goiter regions in the world where iodine is largely lacking—in the Himalayas in Asia, regions of the Alps and Carpathian and Pyrenees mountains in Europe, the high plateaus of the Andes in South America, and in the Great Lakes basin and area of the St. Lawrence River in North America.

In some of these areas in the past, goiter incidence was staggering. It approached 100 percent in the Alpine regions. Never that high in the United States, it nevertheless caused worry in the past. As late as 1936, the Wisconsin State Medical Society's Commission on Goiter found that of 554,000 schoolchildren in the state, 100,000 showed an abnormal thyroid gland. In more recent times, the use of iodized salt has made goiter far less of a problem.

But hypothyroidism can occur—and commonly does—without goiter. And it can result from other than lack of iodine. Other causes include failure to trap iodine in the gland; failure to convert it into usable form; inability to couple other materials into effective hormones.

Overlooked hypothyroidism

Nobody really knows how common hypothyroidism may be. But for many years there have been allegations that it is quite common, much more so than generally realized by physicians as well as the public, and commonly overlooked, particularly in its less than extreme forms.

For one thing, many tests for thyroid function have worked well for the more severe gland disturbances but not always for the mild.

There have also been many charges of a basic confusion within the medical profession about hypothyroidism.

As far back as 1933, Dr. O. P. Kimball, after a ten-year study carried out in part at the Cleveland Clinic and in part in his private practice, was reporting that "in the practice of medicine today no more important condition is encountered or so often unrecognized as such as hypothyroidism." Kimball pointed out that a prime reason for this was a theory that hypothyroidism could not exist without myxedema. On the face of it, the theory made little sense since it presupposed that there could be no milder degrees of thyroid underfunctioning, only a failure so great as to produce extreme symptoms.

Yet this, Kimball noted, was the theory he had been taught as a medical student, and he went on to add: "Just why this teaching should persist now in the face of all the experimental evidence to the contrary is hard to understand."

Half a dozen years later, Dr. G. K. Wharton of the University of Western Ontario published another report that decried essentially the same failing. "Many patients who could be helped by thyroid treatment are not recognized as hypothyroid. Cretinism and myxedema are the textbook examples of the hypofunctioning thyroid gland. Very little has been written about the milder degrees and the atypical forms of deficient thyroid activity. Hypothyroidism in a mild or masked form differs so greatly from myxedema and cretinism that constant alertness for its many and varied manifestations is demanded."

Still many years later, Dr. Arnold Jackson was trying, in a report in the *Journal of the American Medical Association*, to focus medical attention on the fact that "hypothyroidism is the most frequent chronic affliction and at the same time the most overlooked condition affecting persons residing in the Middle West. This statement is based upon an experience of 37 years in diagnosing and treating thousands of these cases seen at the Mayo and Jackson Clinics."

And only very recently, late in the 1970's, Dr. Lewis C. Mills, professor of medicine, Division of Endocrinology and Metabolism, Hahnemann Medical College, Philadelphia, was pointing out that "although patients with severe hypothyroidism or myxedema are readily diagnosed, early or borderline cases often go undetected and therefore are not treated."

Certainly, the symptoms of extreme hypothyroidism are virtually unmistakable. We've touched on them only briefly before. Cretinism, occurring in infants and children as the result of gross thyroid deficiency during fetal or early life, with the gland greatly reduced in size or even entirely absent, produces thick, dry, wrinkled, and sallow skin; enlarged tongue; thickened lips; an open, drooling mouth; a broad face, flat nose, puffy hands and feet. The child is apathetic, dull, and, if untreated, becomes small for his age and a dwarf in adulthood.

Myxedema, the reaction in adulthood to gross thyroid deficiency, resulting from wasting away of the gland, its surgical removal, or failure of the pituitary to stimulate thyroid activity, brings marked physical and personality changes. They include a general, progressive slowing of mental and physical activities, increase in weight, decrease in appetite, a masklike facial appearance, and thickening and rigidity of the skin, which also becomes dry, cold, rough, and scaly. The upper eyelids become waterlogged and the eyebrows elevated in efforts to keep the eyes open. The hair becomes coarse, brittle, and tends to fall out. There is sensitivity to cold with feelings of chilliness in rooms of normal temperature. Many myxedematous patients are troubled by joint pains and stiffness and reduced resistance to infection. They appear slow, drowsy, placid; have difficulty maintaining normal mental effort; tend to drop off to sleep during the day. Depression and decline in sexual function and libido are common. Yet all these manifestations can be controlled when thyroid is administered in suitable dosage.

As cretinism and myxedema indicate, virtually no body system may escape the effects of severe thyroid deficiency. Yet even in the extreme forms of hypothyroidism, there can be variations in manifestations, some being more obvious and troublesome than others.

When hypothyroidism is milder in degree, it can be much more subtle. It, too, may affect many systems, though not all to the same degree. One patient may have manifestations that another does not. It is as if there are variations among individuals in the organs and systems that are most susceptible to thyroid deficiency, variations similar to those among allergic persons in whom sensitivity to a food, pollen, or other material may produce varying symptoms depending upon the "target" organs affected: nasal congestion, discharge, and sneezing when the nose is the target organ; rash, hives, or eczema when the skin is affected; wheezing when the bronchial tubes are particularly sensitive.

Obviously, hypothyroidism is hardly the reason for every mental or mental/physical problem. But with its ability to provoke a wide variety of symptoms, it deserves consideration in many cases.

At the University of North Carolina, Dr. P. C. Whybrow and other investigators, studying a group of patients with mental disturbances who proved to be hypothyroid, found that almost all complained of poor recent memory and difficulty in concentration. Several women complained they no longer could remember cooking recipes they had used for many years. One reported having to depend on her children to remember where she placed things around the house. When tested with simple dollars-and-cents arithmetic problems, many patients had great difficulty.

Some had more serious problems. One woman had come to believe herself a burden to her family and had frequent thoughts of suicide. Preoccupied with memories of a son killed in a car accident years before, she wished she had been the one killed, and dreamed of digging him from his grave with her bare hands and kept hearing his voice calling her during the day.

Another woman had great difficulty sleeping, and when she did sleep, she had morbid dreams that she believed in intensely. She dreamed of her only son dying and of other family members suffering mutilation. She was increasingly worried about losing her mind.

Although these were patients who could easily have been regarded as suffering from severe psychiatric illnesses, their physicians—alert, investigative psychiatrists—checked thyroid function and used thyroid therapy to relieve their illnesses.

At Georgetown University, a study of more than one hundred patients with thyroid underfunctioning showed that inability to concentrate was a prominent symptom in 31 percent, forgetfulness in 26 percent, deafness in 17 percent, ear noises in 8 percent, and poor muscular coordination in another 8 percent. Moreover, abnormal sensations of prickling, tingling, or creeping on the skin were present in 79 percent.

One study reported from the Mayo Clinic by a neurological team headed by Dr. G. M. Cremer covered five men and nineteen women who had been referred for neurological investigation because of puzzling symptoms and who proved to be hypothyroid. The symptoms included mental slowing, poor equilibrium, incoordination of the limbs, muscle disturbances, hearing problems, and abnormal sensations. The symptoms responded to thyroid therapy.

Among the patients was a woman who had been referred for neurological work-up because of suspicion of a brain tumor. She had long experienced episodes of dizziness and, more recently, had also suffered from light-headedness and increased hearing loss. Tests also revealed mental slowing and muscle disturbances. On thyroid treatment, she was able, within two weeks, to walk without dizziness; within six months, normal hearing had returned; at eighteen months, she was completely well.

Dr. Broda O. Barnes of Fort Collins, Colorado, who has spent much of his professional life working with hypothyroid patients, writes in his book *Hypothyroidism: The Unsuspected Illness* of a conviction that as many as 40 percent of Americans today are affected by some degree of hypothyroidism. "They include," he remarks, "many being fed stimulants, tranquilizers or other medications which serve only to somewhat dampen symptoms without getting at the cause. They include many who are considered neurotics or hypochondriacs."

A simple home test

Barnes has developed a simple test which, in his experience, can provide a valuable indication of the possibility of hypothyroidism and can be taken at home.

Called a basal temperature test, it is not generally accepted by physicians as being a precise indication. Nevertheless, it could be useful in a suggestive way, alerting a patient to the need for a careful medical check of thyroid function.

The test involves only one simple piece of equipment—an ordinary thermometer. Shaken down well the night before and placed within arm's reach of the bed, it's used immediately upon awakening in the morning before leaving bed. The thermometer is placed snugly in an armpit for ten minutes by the clock.

The normal range of armpit temperature is 97.8° to 98.2°. A reading below that range suggests low thyroid function. And all the more so if a similar reading is obtained another morning.

The test can be taken by a man on any day. Not so for a woman. During the menstrual years, as women know, temperature fluctuates during the cycle, peaking shortly before the start of flow and reaching its lowest point at the time of ovulation. During the menstrual years, basal temperature is best measured on the second and third days of the period after flow starts. After menopause, it may be measured on any day.

Parathyroid problems

You may recall the woman mentioned briefly in Chapter 3 who for fifteen years had been treated for severe, sometimes suicidal depression with antidepressant drugs and electroshock, until finally her real problem, hyperparathyroidism, was uncovered.

The parathyroid glands secrete a hormone that is a key factor in controlling how the body handles the minerals calcium and phosphorus.

Calcium is the most abundant mineral in the body. In combination with phosphorus it forms calcium phosphate, the dense, hard material of the bones and teeth.

Additionally, a constant level of calcium is required in the blood for many important body functions, including maintenance of the heartbeat, clotting of blood, and normal functioning of muscles and nerves.

In hyperparathyroidism, the excess activity of the glands and their oversecretion of parathyroid hormone lead to elevated levels of calcium in the blood, and this hypercalcemia, or calcium excess, produces symptoms.

Hypercalcemia can lead to weakness, appetite loss, nausea, constipation, abdominal pain, thirst, and excessive urination. Calcium stones may form in the urinary tract. In some cases, bone disease or kidney damage may develop.

In severe hypercalcemia, mental symptoms may include retardation, spells of unconsciousness, delusions, confusion, hallucinations, and memory impairment. With lesser degrees of hypercalcemia, what seem to be psychoneurotic disturbances can occur and may include lassitude, lack of initiative, interest, and spontaneity, and depression.

Hyperparathyroidism most often results from overgrowth of one or more of the parathyroids or from a benign tumor of one of the glands. It is sometimes possible for a tumor of lung or kidney to secrete a compound that has some similarity to parathyroid hormone, causing hypercalcemia. And other possible causes include very severe hyperthyroidism and vitamin D poisoning from excess intake.

Blood tests to measure calcium levels in blood and urine have been available. There is now a highly sensitive blood test, an immunoassay of parathyroid hormone itself, which is valuable not only in diagnosing hyperparathyroidism but even in helping to point to the possible cause.

Effective treatment is the surgical removal of a parathyroid tumor when one is present or the removal of some of the parathyroid tissue when overgrowth is the problem.

The reverse condition of hypoparathyroidism, in which the glands fail to produce adequate amounts of parathyroid hormone and blood levels of calcium are low, can also produce both physical and mental symptoms.

Hypoparathyroidism may occur as the result of accidental removal of or damage to the parathyroid glands during thyroid surgery. In such cases, it becomes obvious within twenty-four hours. There is also a form of hypoparathyroidism called idiopathic, in which the glands are usually absent or wasted, but this is rare. And there is still another form, called pseudohypoparathyroidism, in which there is no deficiency of parathyroid hormone; instead, the hormone is not normally effective.

With hypoparathyroidism, blood levels of calcium are low. When they are very low, the result is tetany, of which the most obvious sign is spasm of the muscles, especially those of fingers and toes. But spasms, or involuntary contractions, may occur in virtually any muscle, including the muscles of face, eyes, tongue, and larynx, or voice box.

In idiopathic hypoparathyroidism, about one-third of patients are intellectually impaired, some to the point of mental retardation. Another third exhibit neuroses and emotional disturbances, including emotional lability, anxiety, depression, and irritability. Such problems are seldom seen in patients with surgically induced hypoparathyroidism, possibly because treatment is usually started immediately.

Treatment is effective. It involves increasing intake of calcium, and a calcium supplement such as calcium gluconate or calcium carbonate may be used. It also calls for suitable doses of vitamin D. The vitamin has actions somewhat similar to those of parathyroid hormone and helps to raise blood calcium to normal levels. It must be properly used in order to avoid vitamin D intoxication and severe hypercalcemia.

Adrenal gland disorders

Let the adrenal glands become underactive, as they do in Addison's disease, or overactive, as they do in Cushing's, and they can produce not only many physical disturbances but emotional and behavioral ones as well, and, in some cases, the latter may be the first to become of concern.

And still another adrenal disorder called a pheochromocytoma, which involves a tumor of an adrenal gland which is usually benign, can also produce both types of disturbances.

The adrenals atop the kidneys play many vital roles in the body economy. Each adrenal is actually a gland within a gland, an outer shell called the cortex and an inner core known as the medulla.

The medulla produces two hormones, epinephrine (adrenaline) and norepinephrine (noradrenaline), which have somewhat similar actions. They influence heart rate, motility in the gastrointestinal tract, and dilation of the pupil of the eye.

The cortex produces many hormones, so many, in fact, that they are divided into three groups: glucocorticoids (cortisol, or hydrocortisone, cortisone, and corticosterone); mineralocorticoids (aldosterone and desoxycorticosterone, and corticosterone); and androgens, or male sex hormones. Also present in adrenal secretions are small amounts of the female sex hormones, estrogen and progesterone. The glucocorticoids help control the body's handling of proteins, fats, and carbohydrates; the mineralocorticoids influence the concentration of sodium and potassium in body fluids.

Addison's disease

This is an insidious, progressive disease in which the adrenal cortex underfunctions. In more than two-thirds of cases, there is a shriveling of the cortex, with cause unknown. In the remainder there is partial destruction, which may be due to inflammation, a disease such as tuberculosis, or malignancy. Addison's disease can occur at any age and affects both sexes equally.

Weakness and fatigue are among the early symptoms. Weight loss, loss of appetite, nausea, vomiting, and diarrhea often occur; sometimes, too, decreased tolerance to cold and episodes of dizziness and fainting. And there may be seemingly psychiatric symptoms—apathy, depression, lack of interest and initiative, poverty of thought, and general negativism.

Skin pigmentation is usually increased and manifested as tanning of both exposed and nonexposed parts of the body. And there may be black freckles over face, forehead, neck, and shoulders and bluish-black discolorations of the lips, mouth, rectum, and vagina.

The diagnosis of Addison's disease is usually suspected when increased skin pigmentation is found, although in some cases this may be minimal.

There are useful tests for uncovering the disease. One in common use involves infusion into a vein of a dose of ACTH, a pituitary hormone that ordinarily stimulates the adrenal glands. If, following an infusion, levels of adrenal hormones in the blood do not rise (in normal people, they double), the test points to Addison's.

Even prior to such a special test, various laboratory findings can suggest Addison's disease. They include blood tests which show a low white blood cell count, an increase in the blood elements called eosinophils, low blood levels of sodium and high levels of potassium. X-ray evidence of a small heart and calcifications in the adrenal areas is also suggestive.

Once Addison's is diagnosed, it can be treated so effectively with hormones to make up for the adrenal cortex's underfunctioning that a patient with even relatively severe disease can expect to lead a full life.

Cushing's syndrome

In this condition, a complex of symptoms may arise from overactivity of the adrenal cortices. The overactivity may be the result of abnormal growth of the cortices or may be caused by a benign or malignant growth of one of the adrenal glands. In some cases, the adrenal overactivity may be stimulated by secretions from a pituitary gland or ovarian tumor.

The symptoms of Cushing's syndrome can include a moonlike fullness of the face, accumulations of fat in the trunk and on the back (buffalo hump), thin skin that is easily bruised, and sometimes purple marks on the abdomen. There may also be general weakness, high blood pressure, abdominal distention, impairment of sexual function, and unusual growth of body hair. Women usually have menstrual irregularities.

Psychiatric disturbances are common. Depression is the most frequent manifestation and as many as 10 percent of patients attempt suicide. Up to 20 percent of patients may even be considered psychotic. Other psychological manifestations can include irritability, difficulty in concentrating, insomnia, paranoid delusions, hallucinations, and, less often, apathy, excitement, anxiety, delirium, disorientation, or loss of recent memory.

The range of mental disturbances is bizarre. And there is some evidence now that the disturbances may differ depending upon the cause of the adrenal overactivity. When the problem lies with excessive stimulation by the pituitary, for example, pituitary as well as adrenal hormones are elevated and the pituitary hormone excess may play a role. When the problem lies with the adrenals without stimulation from the pituitary, adrenal hormones are elevated but pituitary hormones are not.

For diagnosis, blood and urine tests can be used to determine hormone levels. Infusing the pituitary hormone ACTH can help to distinguish between some causes. Skull X-rays for signs of a pituitary tumor and still other tests aid in pinpointing cause.

Treatment, of course, is directed at correcting the overfunctioning of the pituitary gland or the adrenal cortex. Sometimes, irradiation of the pituitary is adequate. In other cases, adrenal gland surgery may be required.

Very recently, promising results have been obtained with a drug, cyproheptadine. Although it is an antihistamine sometimes used for hay fever and other allergies, cyproheptadine has other actions as well. In about 60 percent of patients with Cushing's syndrome for whom the drug has been tried, it has been effective in eliminating symptoms. Its continuous use is needed.

Pheochromocytoma

This, as we noted earlier, is a tumor, usually benign, of an adrenal gland. It occurs in the adrenal medulla. And because it is composed of cells similar to the hormone-secreting cells of the medulla, it is capable of secreting epinephrine and norepinephrine. The symptoms of pheochromocytoma are related to the excessive amounts of such hormones in the tissues and blood.

Almost invariably, the tumor produces high blood pressure, which may be either paroxysmal or persistent. Other symptoms often include severe headache, flushing, cold and clammy skin, chest pain, palpitation, nausea and vomiting, visual disturbances, breathing difficulty, and constipation. Commonly, there is a feeling of great apprehension and a sense of impending doom. And in some cases, the first manifestation of pheochromocytoma may be anxiety for which a patient may seek psychiatric help.

Blood and urine tests help in diagnosis. X-ray and other studies also may be used. Treatment is the surgical removal of the tumor.

Hypopituitarism

When pituitary gland functioning is deficient, behavioral disturbances are likely. Patients with pituitary failure may become dependent, apathetic, depressed, drowsy. They may lose their drive and initiative. Commonly, they are fatigued. Mental effects sometimes can be profound, ranging from confusion to frank psychosis.

The pituitary is divided into two major parts, each producing a number of different hormones. The anterior, or front, lobe produces at least seven hormones. One, growth hormone (HGH), acts directly on tissues of the body to insure proper growth and development of the skeleton. The other six hormones have their primary action on other endocrine glands.

One of the six, thyrotropin, also called thyroid-stimulating hormone (TSH), controls the secretion of thyroid hormone by the thyroid gland. ACTH (adrenocorticotrophic hormone) stimulates the cortex of the adrenal gland to secrete its hormones.

A third anterior pituitary hormone, called follicle-stimulating hormone (FSH), affects the reproductive organs. In women, it stimulates growth of the ovarian follicle and secretion of estrogen; in men, it helps to regulate the formation of spermatozoa. Because it affects the gonads, or sex organs, FSH is also called a gonadotropic hormone. Another gonadotropic hormone is luteinizing hormone (LH). In the female, LH acts with FSH to bring about maturation of the ovarian follicle and also initiates rupture of the mature follicle so that the ovum, or egg, is released. In addition, LH acts upon the cells of the capsule surrounding the follicle with the end result being the production of the hormone progesterone, which is required for pregnancy. In the male, LH is known also as interstitial-cell-stimulating hormone because it stimulates the development of interstitial cells of the testes and thus controls the production of the male sex hormone testosterone.

Still another anterior pituitary hormone, lactogenic or luteotropic hormone (LTH), also known as prolactin and mammotropin, stimulates production of milk in the mammary glands. Melanocyte-stimulating hormone (MSH) is believed to influence formation or deposition of melanin, a dark pigment normally found in hair, skin, eyes, and some nerve cells.

The posterior, or back, lobe of the pituitary produces two hormones. One, vasopressin or antidiuretic hormone (ADH), decreases the rate of urine formation by stimulating reabsorption of water by the kidneys, and is important in maintaining the body's fluid balance; it also increases blood pressure, stimulates contraction of intestinal muscles, and influences the uterus. Underproduction of ADH results in excessive urination and can lead to the relatively rare disorder called diabetes insipidus, not related at all to the more common diabetes mellitus.

In diabetes insipidus, there is not, as in diabetes mellitus, any elevation of sugar in the blood or urine. Instead, large volumes of dilute but otherwise normal urine are excreted. The total volume may reach several gallons a day, and because of the huge loss of water in the urine, there is excessive thirst and need to drink large quantities of water. The use of vasopressin as a nasal spray or an injection corrects the problem.

The second hormone produced by the posterior lobe is oxytocin, which is required for contraction of the uterus during labor and delivery. It is also secreted during nursing and causes ejection of milk from the mammary glands.

Hypopituitarism has many possible causes. It may result from a tumor of the pituitary or from hemorrhage or shock following childbirth. It may also be due to fungal or other infections that spread to the pituitary. In some cases, the ballooning out (aneurysm) of an artery feeding the brain may be responsible.

Depending upon the cause and the degree of effect on the pituitary, one or many or all pituitary hormones may be deficient. TSH deficiency will lead to hypothyroidism and ACTH deficiency to adrenal gland deficiency, with the symptoms already noted for those problems. Lack of FSH and LH can lead to infertility and absence of menses in a woman and to infertility and wasting of the testes in a man. HGH deficiency, perhaps in conjunction with lack of the hormone cortisol from the adrenals, may lead to hypoglycemia, or low blood sugar.

X-rays of the pituitary can be used to determine if a tumor is present. And other tests can be used to try to determine the cause of the hypopituitarism. In addition, tests can be carried out for thyroid, adrenal, and other gland functioning.

Treatment, of course, is directed at the cause. If a pituitary tumor is present, it may yield to irradiation or, when necessary, to surgical removal. Treatment also may involve replacing the hormones of the underfunctioning target glands. Hypothyroidism can be treated with thyroid preparations; adrenal insufficiency with hydrocortisone; hypogonadism in the male can be treated with testosterone preparations and in the female with estrogen preparations.

It is not clear whether the personality changes that occur in hypopituitarism result primarily from adrenal gland failure, thyroid failure, or gonadal failure, or a combination. But adrenal gland failure appears to be important and even crucial since treatment with adrenal steroid hormones alone often will reverse the personality changes. For restoration of libido, however, sex hormone replacement is required. Sex hormones improve libido but have little effect on such other symptoms as lassitude, apathy, indifference, and confusion.

Diabetes

The well-known, common form of diabetes—diabetes mellitus—results when the islet cells in the pancreas fail to produce adequate amounts of the hormone insulin or the insulin fails to act effectively. Without adequate or effective insulin, the body's handling of carbohydrates and other dietary materials is impaired and blood sugar (glucose) levels rise.

Diabetes is known to affect upward of 3.5 million Americans in whom the disorder has been diagnosed. But at least 1.5 million are as yet undiagnosed. The disease is more frequent in women than in men and the incidence increases with age.

The classical symptoms of diabetes are excessive thirst, excessive urination, and excessive hunger. Tendencies toward frequent skin disorders, especially boils, and vaginal infections are common.

Diabetes can also be responsible for many other disturbances: generalized weakness and lassitude, blurring of vision, numbness, tingling, leg cramps, and impotence.

Undetected diabetes also may produce symptoms of anxiety, schizophrenia-like manifestations, and even acute psychotic episodes, and sometimes these may be the first manifestations of the disorder. If recognized for what they are, they can be overcome by medical treatment for the diabetes.

When diabetes is suspected, diagnosis is easily made by measuring the glucose, or sugar, level in the blood. Diet, exercise, and medication can be used in treatment. In mild diabetes, suitable diet and regular exercise are often enough.

The goal of the diet is to bring body weight to an ideal level (especially in adulthood, diabetes is more likely to occur in overweight people), to supply balanced nutrition, and to restrict carbohydrates (especially refined carbohydrates in the form of refined sugar and concentrated sweets), which are poorly handled in the diabetic. Exercise is valuable because it promotes use of blood sugar in muscles.

When diet and exercise are inadequate to control the symptoms of diabetes, insulin may be used or in some cases an oral blood-sugar-lowering drug may be employed.

9. *Mystifying Symptoms and Sometimes Hidden Sleep Disturbances*

A middle-aged Connecticut man not long ago found help for a problem that had plagued him ever since his high-school days. Although he had no trouble falling asleep at night or, to his knowledge, staying asleep for a full eight hours, he woke in the morning exhausted. All during the day he continued to feel exhausted, experienced repeated fits of drowsiness, and was irritable and short-tempered with family and co-workers. He had spent thousands of dollars going from physician to physician seeking help without finding it.

Then he spent one night at a sleep-wake clinic at Montefiore Hospital and Medical Center in The Bronx, New York. There, his problem quickly became obvious as his sleep was monitored with electronic equipment and was video-taped. Hundreds of times during the night he would stop breathing, gasp for air with a loud snore, then resume breathing again. The breathing interruptions were so brief that when he woke in the morning he had no recollection of them.

His treatable problem is called sleep apnea. Long unrecognized, it is estimated to affect at least fifty thousand Americans.

All told, sleep disorders, which include many others in

addition to insomnia, affect millions. Although the true incidence is not known, some surveys have suggested that at least 20 percent of the population suffer from some difficulty related to sleep.

Certainly, emotional disturbances account for sleep problems in many cases. But it is also true that sleep problems may sometimes produce emotional upsets, and that disorders of sleep often may go unrecognized for what they are while the symptoms they produce may be attributed to psychogenic causes.

Very recently, what is coming to be looked upon as almost a new branch of medicine—based on research in special sleep laboratories and clinics—has begun to provide valuable new diagnostic tools and effective treatment methods.

The need for sleep

Obviously enough, sleep is essential, a biologic necessity. Without it, we feel not only physically fatigued but also emotionally drained.

The longest a person can go without sleep, various studies have found, is about 240 hours, or 10 days. And volunteers staying awake that long have found the experience a torture. Even after 65 hours without sleep, one volunteer was discovered in a washroom, frantically trying to wash nonexistent "cobwebs" off his face, convinced he was covered with them.

Although it is generally assumed that eight hours of sleep is the norm, scientific studies have revealed a wide range of requirements. One in Scotland, for example, found that 8 percent of a large sample needed five hours at most, and some got along with less. Fifteen percent needed five to six hours. The majority needed seven to eight hours. But 13 percent required nine to ten, and a few needed even more than ten.

There have been suggestions that body type may be a factor in determining how much sleep is needed, that the endomorph—the soft, fat type of person—sleeps easily and a lot, while the ectomorph—sensitive and fragile—is prone to insomnia. But no definitive studies support the idea.

Some indication that sleep habits may reflect personality traits comes from studies of long and short sleepers by Dr. Ernest L. Hartmann and his colleagues at the Boston State Hospital Sleep Laboratory.

In the laboratory over an eight-night period, twenty-nine volunteers, some who habitually slept less than six hours and others who habitually slept more than eight hours, were given varied psychological and other tests and their sleep was electronically monitored.

Overall, the short sleepers, the Boston investigators found, were more socially adept and dominant in relationships with others. Their vocations included engineering, business, carpentry, contracting. They tended to be conformists, establishment-oriented in job preferences and opinions. They kept busy, tended to avoid psychological problems rather than face them.

Long sleepers had a greater variety of professions and interests. Many held responsible jobs, some were artists, a few were described as "hippies." They were less conformist; some were very creative. But many were shy, some were mildly depressed, and some appeared anxious. Most were somewhat inhibited sexually.

During the study, the long sleepers' sleep was found to contain about twice as much REM, or dream sleep, as the sleep of the short sleepers. Conceivably, they may need to sleep longer and dream more in order to use the greater dream time to resolve psychic problems.

However, some scientists wouldn't be surprised if there were a built-in, genetically determined predisposition for more or less sleep. While training and environment are factors in sleep habits, as they are in eating and other habits, still, as Dr. Julius Segal of the National Institute of Mental Health has observed, "The old phrase, 'born that way,' referring to genetic inheritance, seems increasingly relevant here. That is, the patterns of sleep that many people exhibit or complain about are apparent from earliest childhood.

Many parents who are very upset about a child's sleep patterns ought best to make peace with the fact that these patterns came with the child and are not all that easy to change."

The happenings during sleep

Where once it was thought that sleep was a state of complete oblivion, now it's known to be an up-and-down affair, a composite of at least five distinct cyclic stages.

Two distinct states of sleep, as different from each other as either is from the waking state, can be easily identified. One is REM (rapid eye movement) sleep; the other NREM sleep (without eye movement). And NREM sleep is divided into four stages that range from dozing (stage 1) to deepest sleep (stage 4).

Delicate equipment used in sleep laboratories to detect and amplify brain currents, monitor eye movements, record pulse and breathing rates, body movements, muscle tensions, and other information has shown that as you close your eyes in preparation for sleep, body temperature begins to fall and brain waves show alpha rhythm, a frequency of about nine to thirteen per second. You're still awake but beginning to move into sleep. In stage 1 sleep, the pulse rate slows, muscles relax, and brain waves slow to four to six cycles a second, and this is light sleep.

In stage 2, medium-deep sleep, brain waves grow larger and slower. After about thirty minutes, you move into stage 3, and the waves slow still more. Deepest sleep, stage 4, comes next, but lasts only about twenty minutes, whereupon you begin to move up into lighter sleep again. As you do, you may make some movement, turn in bed, and you reach almost, but not quite, the consciousness level.

Now your eyes begin to move under the closed lids, in much the same fashion as when you watch a movie. And, in fact, at this point, you are dreaming, and if you were to be awakened now, you would recall the dream clearly. After about ten minutes of this rapid eye movement, or dreaming, sleep, you start the whole cycle all over again. Each cycle normally takes about ninety minutes.

That a certain amount of REM sleep is needed has been demonstrated in the laboratory where subjects have been deprived of REM by waking them every time they entered that stage. Later they went through an REM rebound phase in which they spent greater amounts of time in REM and reached the REM state sooner on falling asleep.

Each sleep stage seems to be important and may well serve specific purposes. NREM almost always precedes REM, and some researchers believe that functions carried out during NREM must come before the results are further processed in REM. One theory is that proteins and other substances may be manufactured in the nervous system during NREM and used partly later in REM processes.

Some investigators speculate that stages 3 and 4 of NREM may provide physical rest as well as restore metabolic functions after or in anticipation of high metabolic demands. Vigorous physical exercise late in the day, for example, produces metabolic demands that must be made up by increased amounts of stages 3 and 4 sleep at night, while early-morning exercise does not increase stages 3 and 4 sleep times the following night.

Dr. Ernest L. Hartmann of Boston State has developed a theory that various proteins—structural, enzyme and hormone—produced during NREM sleep may be used during REM to restore nerve cell membrane efficiencies, preparing them for renewed mental activity on waking. The theory suggests that REM is needed to maintain emotional stability in a changing environment.

Sleep apnea

Sleep apnea, in which there are frequent cessations of breathing during sleep that may last from 20 to 130 seconds, has only recently come in for attention, thanks to the ability of sleep laboratories to detect it with special equipment.

And, in fact, out of the laboratory work have come guidelines for physicians that may even be useful to some victims of apnea in suspecting the condition.

At Stanford University School of Medicine, Stanford, California, Dr. Christian Guilleminault and a team of investigators recently reported on a series of twenty-five men aged 25 to 65 in whom apnea was diagnosed after sleep studies.

From their experience, the Stanford physicians note, sleep apnea should be especially suspected in the presence—along with loud snoring—of any of a group of symptoms: abnormal movements during sleep, excessive daytime sleepiness, hallucinations, automatic behavior, personality changes with abnormal behavioral outbursts, even high blood pressure or bed-wetting.

Apneas are classified as either central, upper airway obstructive, or mixed. In central apnea there is a fleeting halt in the regular movement of the diaphragm, the dome-shaped muscle that separates the chest and abdomen and is active in breathing. In upper airway obstructive apnea, there is a collapse of tissue structures of the upper airway, obstructing the airway and preventing breathing although the diaphragm contracts to take a breath. Mixed apnea is a central followed by an upper airway obstructive apnea.

Because apnea may cause several hundred brief or sometimes prolonged arousals during a night, it can be responsible for significant insomnia. The patient, usually unaware of having the apneic episodes, may complain of insomnia or disturbed sleep. Apnea also may cause sleepers to spend all their time in light stage 1 or 2 NREM sleep so they do not get enough stages 3 and 4 sleep. Such sleepers complain of excessive daytime sleepiness and sleep attacks and are diagnosed as hypersomniacs with sleep apnea.

Apneic hypersomnia is sometimes associated with obesity and, when severe, may develop into the Pickwickian syndrome. This is a condition in which the patient experiences upper airway obstructive sleep apnea which leads not only to excessive daytime sleepiness and sleep attacks, but, in addition, there is chronic insufficient breathing (hypoventilation) and therefore low blood oxygen content (hypoxia). And in efforts to overcome the inadequate oxygen supply, the right side of the heart, which pumps blood to the lungs to be oxygenated, works harder and enlarges, pulmonary hypertension develops, and the right side of the heart may eventually weaken.

Actually, the estimate that sleep apnea may afflict at least fifty thousand persons in the United States is considered conservative. Because it is now known that apnea often produces high blood pressure, researchers believe that the estimate might go much higher if all hypertensive patients were tested for apnea. In one study, 60 percent of hypersomniac apnea patients were found to have elevated pressure. Also, the growing numbers of people appearing at sleep disorders centers with sleep apnea suggest that the actual incidence may be much higher than the conservative estimate.

In one study, evidence was found to indicate that as many as 5 percent of people complaining of insomnia suffer from sleep apnea and that as many as 20 percent of those complaining of excessive daytime sleepiness may be afflicted. About 85 percent of sleep patients are male, with symptoms most often occurring after the age of 40.

One aid to diagnosing apnea is simply to question the patient's bed partner to determine if the patient snores especially heavily and with snorting. The loud, heavy, snorting snore is the resumption of breathing after an apneic interruption.

Another aid is for a physician to have the patient go to sleep in his office for an hour or so, wearing a breathing gauge. Breathing stoppages of central apnea will show up on the gauge. However, because many central apnea sufferers may sleep several hours without apnea attacks and apnea may even be entirely absent on any one day, the diagnosis is best established or confirmed in a sleep disorders center.

In hypersomniac apnea patients with their excessive daytime sleepiness, another factor may be involved beyond the lack of restful sleep caused by frequent transient arousals. It is possible, investigators believe, that the buildup of carbon dioxide in the blood during the recurring nighttime apnea may blunt the activity of certain body cells, chemoreceptors, that stimulate breathing. As a result, inadequate breathing, or hypoventilation, may persist during the day as the chemoreceptors send inadequate signals for breathing to breathing centers in the brain.

Hypersomniac apnea patients often have many microsleeps during the day—short sleep periods lasting only a few seconds. They find themselves able to perform simple, routine, repetitive tasks, although sleepy, but not complex acts. The frequent microsleeps may also cause periods of inappropriate behavior and amnesia or memory impairment.

Commonly, too, hypersomniac apnea patients are difficult to rouse fully from a night's sleep. When they do awaken, they often seem disoriented as to time and place and these "foggy mind" periods may last as long as an hour.

Overcoming apnea

To combat severe apnea, a simple surgical procedure, tracheostomy, may be used. A small opening is made in the trachea, or windpipe, area of the throat, and a little tube is inserted in the opening. By day, the patient can plug the tube (which is invisible under collar and tie) and talk normally. By night, with plug removed, the patient inhales through the tube and can sleep soundly without breathing interruption or snoring.

A drug, chlorimipramine, which is now under study and available in the United States only for investigational use, has shown some promise in treating apnea.

The possibility that another medication may help some victims, avoiding need for tracheostomy, has been raised by a finding by Dr. George B. Murray of Massachusetts General Hospital, Boston. Carbamazepine is a drug used for trigeminal neuralgia and other problems unrelated to apnea. Murray prescribed it for a man with another such problem. It worked for that. The patient also turned out to be a victim of apnea and carbamazepine appears to have brought the apnea under control.

Pickwickian syndrome can be treated in part by major weight loss, after which apnea may still occur but less frequently and symptoms of hypersomnia also decrease in intensity. Hormone therapy, either oral progesterone or medroxyprogesterone acetate, is under study as a possible help.

Narcolepsy: "sleepy all the time" and other strange symptoms

Until recently, the 42-year-old wife of a university professor had kept falling asleep during the day, regardless of how well she had slept the night before. Her sleep attacks, sometimes lasting fifteen minutes and occurring frequently, could overpower her suddenly at the dinner table and even when she was driving a car.

Her problem—narcolepsy—is now under control. For her. But not for thousands of other victims.

According to some authorities, the failure to recognize narcolepsy in patients complaining of perplexing chronic fatigue may be the most frequent oversight by physicians.

Because the disorder is unfamiliar to most people as well as to many physicians, an average of fifteen years elapses between its first appearance and diagnosis, says Dr. Christian Guilleminault of Stanford. And according to some informed estimates, two-thirds of victims, who may number in the hundreds of thousands, are undiagnosed.

The narcoleptic attacks

The most characteristic symptom of narcolepsy is what many victims rightly call sleep attacks because they are so overwhelming.

In contrast to excessive daytime sleepiness from other

causes, narcoleptic impulses to sleep are almost irresistible. Sleep has been known to come on even in the midst of a walk or a shower. As many as fifteen to twenty sleep attacks occur daily, each lasting in most cases less than fifteen minutes.

Many victims have another symptom called cataplexy. Some or many body muscles may become suddenly and briefly paralyzed when a strong emotion such as fear or anger is experienced. The face may droop, or there may be a fall to the knees or even a drop to the ground. The eyes may sometimes remain open and the victim is almost always aware of his surroundings during the several seconds to one or two minutes an attack lasts.

A third symptom may be auditory and/or visual hallucinations called hypnagogic hallucinations because they occur at the onset of nighttime sleep or immediately upon waking.

And there may be still a fourth symptom, a fleeting paralysis that occurs at the onset of nighttime sleep or on waking from it. Very briefly, body muscles cannot be moved.

Only a minority of people with narcolepsy experience all four symptoms. In one study of several hundred narcoleptics, all suffered daytime sleep attacks, while 70 percent also had cataplectic attacks. Twenty-five percent experienced hypnagogic hallucinations and 50 percent suffered sleep paralysis. Only 10 percent had all four symptoms.

There seems to be an inherited tendency to narcolepsy. Close relatives of narcoleptics are twenty times more likely than the general population to develop symptoms.

The disorder often begins at puberty, usually as daytime sleep attacks. It has been suggested but not established that the problem may be related to hormonal changes occurring at this stage of development. Cataplexy may not appear for four or five years after sleep attacks begin, and in some cases not until as many as thirty years afterward.

Once established, narcolepsy is lifelong, and unless recognized and treated it can be disabling.

It can handicap a child in school and lead to parent-child misunderstandings and tensions and to emotional troubles.

Drs. Robert E. Yoss and David D. Daly of the Mayo Clinic have described a typical situation in which teachers "may report a decline in the quality of a child's schoolwork, attribute this to inattentiveness which may lead to parental pressure. The child's constant struggle to remain awake in the face of continuing pressure from parents and teachers may cause him to behave impatiently, irritably, suggesting emotional disorder."

Adult sufferers often are stigmatized by relatives, employers, and often by themselves as being "lazy." The stigma may help to account for the incidence of mental depression in 29 percent of one sample of narcoleptics with sleep attacks and in 17 percent more with cataplexy as well. However, some authorities say that the disorder itself may also produce a tendency to depression.

There have been many studies indicating that narcolepsy may be a significant cause of automobile accidents. At the Lahey Clinic in Boston, where for some years narcolepsy has received special study, Drs. Elmer C. Bartels and Osnur Kusakcioglu checked on 105 patients diagnosed at the Clinic as having narcolepsy. They found 81 willing to admit that they had experienced undue drowsiness while driving, 42 who had actually fallen asleep at the wheel, and 17 who had had an accident because they had fallen asleep.

For comparison, the two physicians checked 105 other people without narcolepsy. Only 15 had ever experienced drowsiness while driving, and then only on rare occasions because of inadequate rest. Only one had ever had an accident as the result of falling asleep.

Treatment for narcolepsy

Once diagnosed, narcolepsy can be controlled. The effectiveness of analeptics, drugs that act as central nervous system stimulants, in preventing sleep attacks has been known for many years. The drugs include methylphenidate, pemoline, and dextroamphetamine.

For many victims, treatment with one or another of these

agents has made jobs far easier to handle. Women for whom household chores and raising children once seemed almost insuperable problems have no longer found them problems at all. Many of the successfully treated have reported that their lives have become rewarding in other ways. Going out to dinner, entertaining guests at home, reading, playing cards, watching television, all of which had been burdensome before, have become sources of pleasure.

Children, too, have responded gratifyingly. Among those seen and treated at the Mayo Clinic, for example, was a boy brought there because of queer "spells." He had to lie down several times a day and sleep ten to twenty minutes. He had been seen falling asleep in the midst of play with friends. In school he had fallen asleep repeatedly in class. Between sleep periods, he yawned repeatedly. Placed on methylphenidate, he had no more episodes of abnormal sleepiness.

In one study at the Lahey Clinic of a group of forty-one patients, all previously treated unsuccessfully for "fatigue" thought to be due to a variety of other problems, thirty-eight benefited promptly from analeptic therapy.

Other symptoms of narcolepsy, when present, may be helped by treatment. Drugs such as imipramine and protriptyline may prevent cataplexy. Both are antidepressant agents, but their anticataplectic effect seems unrelated to their antidepressant activity.

Solving the diagnostic problem

The solution to the narcolepsy diagnostic problem often may lie with victims and their families. Diagnosis should not be particularly difficult when all four of the symptoms are present. Such cases are more likely to be diagnosed promptly than others. But all four symptoms occur together in only a minority of narcolepsy victims.

Many who suffer from sleep attacks alone seek no medical help, considering that they have a personal quirk about which nothing can be done. Many who do consult a physician may make diagnosis difficult because of the way they word their complaint.

Narcoleptics often tend to use "fatigue" or other terms—"lack of pep," "lack of energy," "tiredness," "weariness," "listlessness," "no ambition," or "exhaustion"—instead of "irresistible drowsiness" or "irresistible sleep attacks." The terms that patients generally use describe conditions that may stem from many other causes and can be misleading.

If for you or someone in your family, repeated attacks of overpowering sleepiness during the day despite adequate sleep at night is a problem, don't neglect it. See a physician. When you do, describe the problem accurately. The right description is a major help in accurate diagnosis and effective treatment.

When there is any doubt, a sleep clinic can help. All-night sleep monitoring is valuable for clear-cut narcolepsy detection. At night, narcoleptics tend to fall directly into REM sleep while normal people usually do not enter REM until more than ninety minutes after falling asleep.

(Founded by victims of the disorder, the American Narcolepsy Association, Box 5846, Stanford, California 94305, now provides much valuable information for narcoleptics and their families.)

Insomnia: the past confusion

Until very recently, insomnia has gotten the short end of the medical stick.

According to some surveys, about half of all Americans over fifteen years of age have complained about sleeplessness at some time in their lives; about 15 percent say they experience chronic sleeping difficulty; another one-third have more or less recurrent episodes of insomnia.

Although insomnia is a complex problem that can be produced by any of a considerable number of causes and so should have careful diagnosis, too often patients complaining of it have been dismissed with a quick prescription for sleeping pills.

Dr. Ernest L. Hartmann, one of the pioneer sleep investigators, estimates that thirty million Americans currently are taking prescribed or over-the-counter medication to help them sleep. Yet rarely is the medication needed or helpful; sometimes it can aggravate a sleep problem or even produce one where none existed.

"The patient relying on hypnotics [sleeping pills] is often left with his original insomnia plus a drug problem," says Dr. Quentin R. Regestein of the Sleep Clinic of Peter Bent Brigham Hospital, Boston.

Commonly, hypnotic drugs lose their efficacy after only two weeks of use. This may result from the body's increased efficiency in breaking them down, from increased tolerance to their effect developed by the brain, or from other biochemical mechanisms. The patient may become tempted then to increase the dosage because of return of insomnia. Finally, he may become habituated to large doses. He still suffers from poor sleep but must continue use of the drug to get what little sleep he can.

Moreover, hypnotics often suppress REM sleep, during which dreaming occurs. Attempts to stop using a drug lead to an REM rebound—compensatory increased amounts of REM sleep—and may lead to nightmares. In such cases, patients may return to use of the hypnotic to get relief from the nightmares as well as insomnia.

Physicians at Stanford University's Sleep Clinic report that about 40 percent of patients complaining of insomnia actually have sleep problems because they become dependent on the very drugs taken to "treat" their insomnia. And when the drugs are gradually eliminated—carefully, a dose every five or six days, to avoid withdrawal reactions of intense dreams and nightmares—patients average about 20 percent more sleep and many become free of insomnia.

One patient seen at the Stanford clinic had been taking six different sleeping pills, a total of 8,000 milligrams a night, for thirty years and was still "destroyed" by his sleeping problem. It took two years to slowly withdraw him from the pills, after which he was sleeping six and a half hours a night instead of four and a half.

Pseudoinsomnia

Some people get trapped into a pill habit because of what sleep experts call pseudoinsomnia. They have no insomnia problem at all but become convinced they do, sometimes with the help of spouses, because they sleep less than the seven-and-a-half-hour mean normal sleep time.

One investigator tells of a successful professional man who sought help after being convinced by his wife that he was an insomniac because, although both retired at 11 P.M. and she slept through to 6:30 or 7 A.M., he was invariably up at 4:30 or 5 A.M.

Was he tired during the day? Was his "insomnia" interfering with his work or other activities? "Not really," he said reflectively. "I get along fine."

"What's wrong with you," the physician informed him, "is nothing except that you don't need as much sleep as your wife or many other people. And that's hardly a handicap. I have a prescription for you: when you wake up, get up and get going." Which he has done happily since.

Sometimes it takes much convincing before a pseudoinsomniac accepts the fact that there is no problem. Dr. William C. Dement of Stanford has reported that in some cases "cures" are achieved only when patients are shown they are getting adequate sleep according to sleep-recording chart records.

Emotionally induced insomnia

Real insomnia has many possible causes—emotional, physical, and behavioral—and will disappear when causes, rather than the insomnia itself, which is a symptom, are treated.

Certainly, insomnia can stem from emotional disturbances. In some cases, the underlying emotional problem may not be apparent to the patient or even to his physician, according to a study at the Sleep Research and Treatment Center of the University of California at Los Angeles. In the study, which covered 128 people who had become patients at the Center, depression headed the list of emotional problems. Some of the depressed had difficulty falling asleep; others slept a few hours, then were awake the rest of the night.

When depression or another emotional problem such as anxiety is the cause of insomnia, treatment—by antidepressant or other specific medication or possibly in some cases by brief psychotherapy—may be needed. Sleeping pills won't solve the problem.

Some physical causes

Any discomfiting physical problem is capable of causing sleeping difficulty.

Among physical causes of insomnia are insomniac apnea, which we discussed earlier, nocturnal myoclonus, restless legs syndrome, and painful nocturnal erections, which we will be discussing below and which are now being found to be common causes.

Others include allergic diseases such as asthma; painful diseases such as arthritis, ulcers, and nocturnal migraine headaches; neurological disorders such as epilepsy and Parkinson's disease; and metabolic diseases such as diabetes, kidney disease, and hyperthyroidism. Effective control of such diseases may solve the insomnia problem.

For example, Parkinson's disease patients who are not being treated have decreased amounts of total sleep time and of REM sleep, along with frequent wakings. Increased amounts of undisturbed sleep and the normal amount of REM sleep may be restored after treatment of the disease with the anti-Parkinsonism agent L-dopa.

Hyperthyroid patients may have fragmented sleep, low

total sleep time, and a higher-than-normal amount of stages 3 and 4 sleep. Up to a year may be required for normal sleep patterns to be restored after the patient has been rendered euthyroid (normal).

Uneasy legs and insomnia

In as many as 20 percent of chronic insomnia cases, recent studies indicate, the cause is one or another, or a combination, of two strange problems: nocturnal myoclonus and restless legs syndrome.

Nocturnal myoclonus is a jerking movement of the legs every twenty-five to forty seconds during sleep. The jerking motion often arouses the sleeper for five to fifteen seconds. Attacks may last from minutes to several hours during sleep and in severe cases there may be as many as four hundred arousals a night. Patients are usually unaware of the jerking movements. Commonly, however, the sleeping partner can tell stories of being kicked.

The restless legs syndrome makes it difficult or even impossible for its victims to keep their legs still while lying quietly in bed awake. They may also experience uncomfortable, although not painful, creeping sensations deep in the muscles of the lower legs and must often get out of bed to "walk off their legs" for ten to twenty minutes. The delay in finally getting to sleep results in complaints of sleep-onset insomnia.

People with the restless legs syndrome almost always have nocturnal myoclonus as well, although many with nocturnal myoclonus do not have the restless legs syndrome.

In some cases, caffeine may be a contributory factor and its avoidance may be helpful. Diazepam has been used for both conditions with limited success. The drug may decrease the creeping sensations that compel the sleeper to get up and walk around. It is partly effective against myoclonus. In some severe cases, it has reduced the number of wakings to forty or less and also reduced the intensity of the jerks. Carbamazepine, a drug sometimes used in epilepsy and trigeminal neuralgia, has been helpful for the restless legs syndrome.

Dr. Samuel Ayres, Jr., emeritus professor of medicine at UCLA, has found vitamin E of value. The finding was fortuitous. A patient Ayres was treating with the vitamin for a skin problem remarked that since he had begun using it he had stopped having the restless legs problem that had bothered him for years.

With good reason, Ayres became interested. He and his wife were restless legs victims. Both began taking vitamin E with what he has described as "a prompt and gratifying response."

After that, Ayres used it for a series of 134 patients. Of 125 with myoclonus, present in most cases for more than five years, only 2 failed to benefit; 103 had complete relief. Of 9 with restless legs, 7 were completely relieved, the 2 others partially.

Ayres prescribes vitamin E, in the form of d-alpha-tocopheryl acetate or succinate, in doses of 400 international units from one to four times daily before meals, but starts with much smaller doses in patients with high blood pressure or heart problems and in diabetics on insulin. He has reported on his work, for the guidance of physicians, in the *Southern Medical Journal,* Volume 67, page 1308.

Behavioral insomnia

Sleep research is a relatively new area and many aspects of sleep remain to be investigated. One that is beginning to receive attention is the relationship between insomnia and certain customs, habits, and conditionings and how the latter can be corrected.

One leader in such research is Dr. Richard R. Bootzin, a psychologist at Northwestern University, Evanston, Illinois, who considers habitual misuse of the bed to be a common factor in insomnia.

To correct the habit, Bootzin gives patients specific instructions as illustrated in the case of a 25-year-old married man who for more than four years had tried to go to sleep nightly at midnight and had been unable to get to sleep until three or four o'clock in the morning, stewing about various problems to the point where he often turned to reading or watching TV to try to stop stewing.

Bootzin's prescription for him: Go to bed to sleep (sexual relations are another matter) only when you're tired, and once there, no TV, reading, or worrying. Stay in bed to sleep, not to stew. If sleep fails to come within a short time, get out of bed and leave the room. Return to bed only when you're ready to try to fall asleep again. And if you still don't fall asleep soon, get out of bed and leave the room again, and keep repeating the process until you do get to sleep quickly after getting back to bed. No matter if it is a weekday or a weekend and no matter how much sleep you get in a night, set the alarm for the same time every morning. The body needs rest, and a regular schedule will help you get it.

Typically, the patient in this case had to leave the bedroom four and five times a night. But after two weeks of increasingly associating the bedroom with sleep rather than worry, reading, or TV viewing, he was getting two to four hours more sleep each night and at the end of two months was leaving the bedroom no more than once a week.

Other investigators who have used this technique have reported reductions of delays in falling asleep from ninety minutes or more to less than twenty minutes after four weeks.

In some cases, other changes in habits may be required: avoidance of daytime naps; of coffee, tea, or caffeine-containing soft drinks in the evening; of eating the last big meal of the day any later than several hours before bed.

Sleep investigators have also identified a condition called REM intrusion insomnia, in which the sleeper wakes about ninety minutes after falling asleep and continues to awaken throughout the night. In all-night sleep recordings, such people have been found to awaken at the onset of an REM sleep period, during which most dreaming occurs. The theory is that unpleasant dreams over a period of time may have conditioned, or habituated, the sleeper to wake to avoid the REM period. Chlordiazepoxide has been reported to be helpful in breaking the habit.

Still another conditioned insomnia—internal arousal insomnia—has been identified and related to the sleeper's efforts to "will" himself to sleep. This form of sleeping problem may begin with concern to sleep well before important events, and the concern may then become habitual, with continuing efforts to will sleep, during which an internal state of arousal is maintained.

Some investigators have reported success in training such patients in the office in techniques of muscle relaxation, self-hypnosis, or meditation. To show a patient when his relaxation efforts are succeeding, EMG (electromyographic) feedback may be used to amplify and display signals from electrodes placed on the skin over certain muscles. Once successful in achieving effective relaxation with the help of biofeedback, the patient can achieve it in bed without need for equipment.

In some cases, too, bouts of insomnia have been found to lead to a phobia, an unreasonable fear of insomnia, which then establishes the insomnia. Some investigators report success in eliminating the phobia by instructing patients to remain awake at night as long as possible until their need for sleep overpowers the phobia.

Nature's sleeping aid

For some years, some investigators, notably Dr. Ernest L. Hartmann of Boston, have reasoned that there might be some substance, a natural hypnotic, used by the body in producing and regulating sleep.

If such a substance did exist, it would have to be one readily available to the body either from food or through natural body synthesis processes. It would have to be shown, by scientific measurement, to produce a normal night of sleep and to act at doses or concentrations equivalent to those that might occur naturally.

There is evidence now that such a substance has been found in the form of L-tryptophan, a naturally occurring amino acid, one of the building blocks of protein.

L-tryptophan is consumed daily in a normal diet in amounts of 0.5 to 2 grams. In various experimental studies with human subjects, the most common side effect of L-tryptophan proved to be drowsiness.

And in sleep laboratory investigations with people who at home needed fifteen minutes or more before falling asleep, Hartmann and his co-workers found that a dose of 1 gram of L-tryptophan halved the fall-asleep time. Moreover, checking—with all-night records of sleep stages, cycle length, and number of awakenings—showed that L-tryptophan produced normal-appearing sleep.

Sometimes so-called "old wives' tales" turn out to have some validity. And, as Hartmann points out, "the ancient prescription of a glass or two of milk at bedtime may involve more than a psychological 'association to mother.'" For L-tryptophan is present in milk and in other foods, such as meat and green vegetables.

In another test of the ability of L-tryptophan to act as a natural sedative, Dr. Clinton Brown of Johns Hopkins and Dr. Althea M. I. Wagman of the Maryland Psychiatric Research Center in Catonsville, Maryland, chose twelve insomniacs who often spent up to an hour getting to sleep. Over a two-week period, they reported to the Center, where their sleep patterns could be electronically monitored through the night. Before going to bed, they received either tablets of L-tryptophan or, for comparison, an inert placebo.

The study showed that the insomniacs fell asleep twice as fast with L-tryptophan as without it, and slept about forty-five minutes longer than usual without any disturbance in normal stages of sleep.

The possibility of marketing L-tryptophan as a sleeping pill is foreseen by Dr. Wagman, who points out that, in any case, the substance is available in a glass of warm milk to be taken at bedtime.

Hypersomnias

In recent investigations, a whole series of sleep disorders involving excessive daytime sleepiness—disorders other than narcolepsy and sleep apnea—has been identified. Some are very rare; some, relatively more common.

One is the *Kleine-Levin syndrome,* in which there are periods of severe daytime sleepiness along with excessive eating and excessive sex drive. Because male sex hormones can produce a similar condition, some investigators believe that the syndrome may result from overreaction to the hormones by the hypothalamus region of the brain, which may not have matured completely at maturity. Men with the syndrome tend to be young, abnormally shy, and withdrawn. Women can experience the same or a similar condition before onset of an irregular menstrual period. Lithium carbonate has been helpful in preventing attacks in some cases. In women, the symptoms often disappear with the next regular menstrual period or after using an estrogen/progesterone supplement.

In another disorder, called the *subwakefulness syndrome,* despite normal nighttime sleep, sleepiness is present all day and there are frequent periods of microsleep lasting less than a minute each but producing lapses of memory and difficulty in concentration. This rare disorder is apparently the result of a defect of the brain's arousal mechanism involving an insufficiency of a nerve transmitter chemical, dopamine. Investigations are under way to treat victims with dopa (dihydroxyphenylalanine), a compound that is converted to dopamine in the brain.

In still another disorder, called *high 5-HIAA hypersomnia,* abnormally high levels of 5-hydroxyindoleacetic acid (5-HIAA) have been found in the cerebrospinal fluid. The substance, 5-HIAA, is a metabolic material from which another nerve transmitter, serotonin, is formed, and its presence in cerebrospinal fluid in abnormally large amounts may indicate higher amounts of serotonin than normal in the brain. Such patients have been treated successfully with inhibitors of serotonin, such as methysergide.

Isolated sleep paralysis

Although sleep paralysis is a symptom of narcolepsy, it sometimes occurs alone and may be a separate sleep disorder. As in narcoleptic sleep paralysis, the sufferer, for a brief period, is able to move only his eyes and to breathe.

Drug treatment does not seem to be indicated for isolated sleep paralysis. An affected person can will the end of an attack by vigorous movement of the eyeballs and attempts to blink, followed by the moving of facial muscles and then more distant muscles.

Painful nocturnal erections

Penile erections during the night are normal. They occur in 80 to 90 percent of REM sleep periods. In some men, however, even though erection in the waking state is not painful, the nocturnal erections are and often wake the sleeper.

The cause is still unknown and no treatment is known. A reassuring fact is that the painful erections have no effect on normal sexual activity.

Night terror attacks

In night terror, a sleeper suddenly sits up in bed, awakening from sleep, eyes open, pale, with a terrified expression, and screams and moans. After an episode, which may last fifteen to thirty minutes, the patient usually goes right back to sleep and does not remember the incident in the morning.

Night terrors usually occur in childhood, most commonly beginning at age 4 to 5 and ending at about age 7 or 8. However, they sometimes do occur in adults.

Night terrors are not the same as nightmares. Nightmares, which are "bad dreams," occur during REM sleep and can be recalled afterward. Night terrors, however, occur during stage 3 or 4 sleep, the deepest stages of NREM sleep. They may sometimes be associated with sleepwalking, sleep talking, and bed-wetting in children.

Night terrors sometimes occur as a symptom in epilepsy, and in such cases appropriate anticonvulsant medication has been used successfully. Otherwise, when they occur in a child, they are thought to be related to immaturity of the nervous system. And experts advise that parents should be counseled by physicians that the child will probably outgrow the condition, that it is not caused by emotional difficulties, and does not produce any carry-over into waking life.

In adults, night terrors may be caused by emotional problems but need not be. Diazepam is often successful in reducing the incidence of night terrors. The drug, trade named Valium, is a tranquilizer, but it is also known to suppress stages 3 and 4 sleep.

Sleepwalking

Sleep researchers now believe that about 15 percent of all children have sleepwalked at least once. It appears to be an inherited tendency, particularly for males, who comprise most of the chronic sleepwalkers. Adults as well may be affected.

The sleepwalker's eyes may be open but they are glassy and unseeing. While a walker may move about a home, critical judgment may be lacking, so that he may fall over furniture or even through a window.

Walking usually takes place in the first part of the night,

when sleep stages 3 and 4 tend to be predominant. A sleepwalk may be an actual walk for five to thirty minutes or merely sitting up in bed for fifteen to thirty seconds. EEG recordings made of subjects while they have been walking show brain waves typical of stages 3 and 4 sleep; and, because dreams occur during REM sleep, and sleepwalking takes place in NREM sleep, a sleepwalker is not acting out a dream, as long supposed.

Children usually outgrow sleepwalking, and investigators believe the disturbance may be due to immaturity of a child's nervous system. Parents also can be reassured that sleepwalking does not indicate emotional problems and will have no emotional effects on a child's later life.

In adults, frequent sleepwalking may be associated with emotional disturbances but in many cases is not. Both the tranquilizer diazepam and the antidepressant imipramine have been successful in reducing sleepwalking. Chronic use of either drug in children is not recommended. But Dr. Leon Tec of the Mid-Fairfield Child Guidance Center, Norwalk, Connecticut, has reported using 25 to 50 milligrams of imipramine before bedtime in children and adults. The drug benefited both groups, and in both just two weeks of treatment proved to be enough, with medication not required thereafter.

Hypnotic suggestion has also been used to reduce sleepwalking in some adults. Using what amounted to a behavioral modification technique, one wife stopped her husband from sleepwalking by whistling derisively every time he rose from bed. Deep muscle relaxation training with the aid of muscle biofeedback has reduced both high sleeping muscle tension and the frequency of sleepwalking.

Sleep talking

Also known as somniloquy, sleep talking is more common in children than adults and the talk is usually incomprehensible. While frequent, purposeful, understandable sleep talking in adults may sometimes indicate emotional problems, somniloquy in a child does not indicate psychiatric problems and the child is likely to outgrow it. Diazepam has reduced sleep talking frequency.

Bed-wetting

Bed-wetting, or enuresis, as it is known medically, is persistent bed-wetting beyond what seems to be a normal age in children: 4 to 5 years. At that point, most youngsters outgrow the wetting. But enuresis persists in 10 percent or a little more of children up to age 5, in 10 percent at age 7, 3 percent at age 12, and in as many as 3 percent even up to the age range of 17 to 28.

Wetting usually occurs in the first part of the night during NREM sleep, so the wetter is not acting out a dream. If the wetter, however, passes into REM sleep soon after the wetting incident, wetness may be incorporated into a dream, a coincidence that has led to a mistaken association between enuresis and dreaming.

Enuresis is called primary when it persists beyond the normal age and secondary when wetting returns after months or years of continence.

The primary form may be the result of late maturing of the nervous system. But it may have organic causes such as obstruction in a male of the urethra, the canal extending from bladder to outside the body; a displaced ureter, the tube conducting urine from kidney to bladder, in a female; a pouch (diverticulum) in the urethra; epispadias, opening of the urethra into a groove on the upper side of the penis; a fissure, or narrow slit or cleft, in the upper wall of the female urethra; bladder malformation; or bladder infection (cystitis).

In at least some persistent bed-wetters, urinary tract allergy may be responsible. Drs. J. W. Gerrard and A. Zaleski of the University of Saskatchewan, Saskatoon, Canada, have reported a study in which twenty-five children were placed on a diet excluding such common allergenic foods as cow's milk, dairy products, chocolate and cola drinks, eggs, citrus fruits and juices, and tomatoes. Five became completely continent and six others showed marked improvement.

Some children bed-wet because of immature, inadequate bladder capacity. Capacity may be increased by having a child hold his urine as long as he can during the day, encouraging him by keeping a record of the increasing amount of urine he can hold before pressure becomes unbearable.

Use of a blanket that sets off a bell or buzzer and wakes the child when he wets may be helpful. But experts urge that it be used with care and compassion and only under guidance from a behavioral therapist experienced in the technique.

Secondary enuresis may indicate an emotional problem, but it can be caused by diabetes or other disease and this possibility should be investigated.

The antidepressant drug imipramine has been used successfully to reduce enuresis. The drug seems to act not through its antidepressant effect but by reducing bladder stimulation.

Tooth grinding

Also known as bruxism, tooth grinding can be a daytime habit and/or a nighttime sleep disorder. It can wear down the teeth and may cause tooth loss and damage to the gums. At night, bruxism occurs during stage 1 or 2 NREM sleep.

Daytime bruxism has been treated successfully by biofeedback. Sleep bruxism is usually treated by the wearing of rubber tooth guards. A U.S. Army study reported successful treatment of sleep bruxism by biofeedback in 75 percent of a group of soldiers but relapse rates are not known.

Jactatio capitis nocturna

This condition, a rhythmic hitting of the head against a pillow or rocking of the body as a ritual of going to sleep, occurs in some infants and young children.

Although it is considered to be a sleep disorder, it seems to cause no ill effects, does not appear to be a symptom of any neurological disorder, is eventually outgrown, and may be in the same class as thumb-sucking as a comforting habit.

Sleep clinics

Accurate diagnosis of many sleep disorders is often possible for a family physician who is in no rush to dispense sleeping pills or tranquilizers but takes the time to delve deeply into an individual patient's complaint.

When necessary, the physician can refer the patient to a sleep disorders clinic for more thorough evaluation.

The clinic will obtain the patient's medical history together with results of a recently performed physical examination and blood, urine, and other laboratory tests. The clinic may send the patient a diary in which, for several weeks in advance of his clinic visit, he makes detailed entries about his hours of work, sleep, other activities, diet, and any drugs he may be taking.

At the center, physicians review the medical history and perform a general physical and neurological examination. They administer a questionnaire eliciting all details of the sleep disorder and may also use psychological and other tests.

Sleep monitoring studies may then follow. Sometimes, monitoring of a daytime nap is all that is required. In other cases, all-night recordings for several nights may be needed to identify, for example, the type and severity of sleep apnea.

The sleep clinic can establish or rule out the presence of sleep apnea, narcolepsy, or other sleep-disturbing conditions. The clinic can prescribe any useful medication for a diagnosed disorder, withdraw any drug to which the patient has become habituated, and, when necessary for a severe sleep apnea, can recommend or carry out a tracheostomy.

More and more sleep clinics are being set up at university hospitals and major medical centers. Your family physician should have no difficulty in referring you to one. If there should be a problem about finding a nearby clinic, the address of one can be obtained from the American Association of Sleep Disorders Centers, University of Cincinnati Sleep Disorder Center, Christian R. Holmes Hospital, Eden and Bethesda Avenues, Cincinnati, Ohio 45219.

10. Epilepsy in Disguise

One day while being teased by classmates, a shy 13-year-old girl suddenly lashes out with a knife and stabs a little boy. Subsequent investigation reveals that she has a history of more than thirty visits to a local hospital. Her frequent headaches and other physical complaints, however, have been assumed to be psychosomatic. Only after the stabbing is she tested and found to have epilepsy.

A middle-aged man suddenly begins to experience episodes of delirium and "insane" behavior. During the episodes, he seems psychotic, totally divorced from reality. He is diagnosed as being the victim of serious psychiatric disease. But he is not. Although he has had no observable seizures accompanying the episodes, he is finally found to have epilepsy.

Rare cases? No. Untreatable? No.

Epilepsy is a vastly misunderstood problem.

Many people still believe that it is rare, but it afflicts at least two million and possibly as many as four million or more Americans. A more exact estimate of the incidence is difficult because many victims and their families still hide the affliction. Too many people also believe that epilepsy is untreatable, although the fact is that the majority of patients, when properly diagnosed and adequately treated, can lead essentially normal lives.

There is another important source of misunderstanding. In addition to, or instead of, the classical forms of epileptic seizures, epilepsy can be manifested by abnormalities of behavior and thought, by impulsivity and aggressive acts, by illusions and hallucinations, by feelings of depersonalization and unreality, by depression with suicidal impulses, by automatic actions, and by other signs and symptoms that are usually associated with and can be mistaken for psychiatric disorders.

Some experts like to say that there is no disease called epilepsy and that what they may be called upon to treat is a wide range of symptoms caused by sudden massive discharges of electrical activity of the brain that are out of phase with normal electrical activity of the brain and bring on seizures.

Familiar types

The three major forms of epilepsy are grand mal, petit mal, and temporal lobe, which is also known as psychomotor.

The best-known, by far the most dramatic, often frightening to bystanders, is grand mal. The grand mal seizure in its classic form has sometimes been called the "wall-to-wall fit." It is produced when almost all cells in the brain fire rapidly and without coordination.

It may start with a premonition period that may occur from several hours to just several seconds beforehand. There may be some peculiar warning change—nausea, lights flashing, ringing in the ears, a strange tingling warmth in some part of the body, or a disorder of smell or taste.

The seizure itself may start with a groan or loud cry followed by a fall and violent twitching or contorting, which may last one to five minutes. Thereafter, the patient may sleep heavily for several hours.

Petit mal is most common in children. A seizure lasts about ten seconds, rarely more than thirty, without loss of muscle tone or falling. There is a sudden dimming of consciousness, a "blank state" during which the patient stops any activity. Immediately afterward, the activity is resumed. A seizure, often referred to as an "absence," can be so fleeting that it may go undetected. Attacks are likely to occur several or many times a day, often when the patient is sitting quietly.

Psychomotor epilepsy, which affects about one-third of adults who have seizures, is characterized by a brief loss of contact with the environment. It may sometimes be difficult to detect because it may be manifested by seemingly purposeful behavior without the obvious changes found in grand mal. The patient does not fall but in some cases may stagger. In some cases, he may perform automatic, purposeless movements and utter unintelligible sounds. He may not understand what is said and may resist help. He may hear or smell things that are not present. Mental confusion may persist for a minute or two after the one- to two-minute attack is apparently over.

There are many possible causes of seizures. They include brain injury at birth or later in life, brain tumor, infection such as meningitis or encephalitis, disturbances produced by toxic substances such as lead and camphor, toxic reactions to excessive alcohol or drug consumption, hemorrhage or clotting of a blood vessel supplying the brain, fever (usually in a child only), and metabolic disturbances such as low blood calcium or low blood sugar. There is also idiopathic epilepsy, for which no cause is known.

Diagnosis may require a careful history of symptoms and any previous medical problems, a thorough physical examination, and studies that may include measurement of blood sugar and calcium, skull X-rays, and electroencephalogram.

When there is a known cause for seizures, the disorder often is remediable. With the cause eliminated—by correction of low blood sugar or calcium, for example—no further treatment may be required.

In other cases, drug therapy can be employed. Although

drugs do not cure, they serve the important function of helping to prevent excessive activity of susceptible brain cells.

With suitable drug treatment, grand mal seizures can be completely controlled in half of cases and greatly reduced in frequency in another 35 percent; petit mal can be controlled in one-third and frequency reduced in another one-third; and psychomotor attacks can be abolished in about 28 percent and reduced in frequency in another 50 percent.

Some masks of epilepsy

Epilepsy can take puzzling forms.

Sometimes there may be mysterious physical symptoms, as in abdominal epilepsy. Recurring attacks of abdominal pain are common in children and often no usual cause for them can be found. In some cases, epilepsy may be responsible. Typically, abdominal epilepsy—which, although largely a childhood manifestation, may sometimes occur in adults—produces attacks of mid- or upper-abdominal pain lasting no more than a few minutes, sometimes accompanied by nausea, vomiting, and appetite loss, and by some confusion but no seizure or loss of consciousness. Usually, after an episode, the patient falls asleep and, upon awakening, feels well.

Recent reports indicate that the great majority of patients with abdominal epilepsy can be freed of symptoms with an anticonvulsant agent such as diphenylhydantoin, and, in fact, a positive response to such a drug can help to confirm the diagnosis of abdominal epilepsy.

Epilepsy also can be responsible for extreme behavioral disturbances. Dr. Charles E. Wells of Vanderbilt University, Nashville, reported recently on a study of a series of patients ranging in age from 10 to 75 years. All had experienced episodes of delirium and psychotic behavior. All had been diagnosed, mistakenly, as having serious psychiatric disorders.

In none of these patients were psychotic episodes accompanied by observable seizures. Yet all proved to have epilepsy and the psychotic episodes could be controlled by long-term treatment with anticonvulsant drugs.

Suggests Dr. Wells: Such psychosis, which can be called ictal psychosis (ictal meaning characterized by sudden attack), should be suspected when any one or more of the following are present: abrupt onset of psychotic behavior in a previously healthy person; unexplained delirium; a history of similar episodes with sudden exacerbations and improvements; a history of fainting or falling spells.

Petit mal as a fooler

Among epilepsy experts, it is believed that some children who have been "diagnosed" by teachers, parents, or other people as lazy, inattentive, and learning-disabled are in reality suffering from undiagnosed petit mal.

Moreover, it now appears that petit mal may sometimes do more than produce "absence" seizures. Several cases have been reported recently in which depression of a serious nature, involving withdrawal, veiled hostility, and suicidal thoughts, was accompanied by the typical EEG, or brain wave, pattern of petit mal. And although petit mal is often said not to start up in late life, the cases of depression occurred in adults.

Grand mal beyond convulsions

Grand mal epilepsy, too, can produce psychiatric symptoms. Confusional states, psychotic states, and prolonged twilight states may occur. Twilight states may consist of any of a variety of disturbances: disorientation, aimless wandering, lip smacking and chewing movements, searching movements of head and eyes. And the psychiatric symptoms may develop in addition to, or instead of, obvious convulsions.

One recently reported example of grand mal epilepsy

with predominantly psychiatric symptoms was a young married woman who was brought to a hospital emergency room in Tucson, Arizona, by her mother because of strange actions that had been going on for a week.

The emergency room physician, who examined her quickly, requested a psychiatric consultation. The psychiatrist found the woman unresponsive to questioning, although she seemed to want to reply. In fact, because she wanted to answer the questions and could not, she tried to leave but was easily brought back.

When she was asked whether she was having difficulty thinking, she nodded. The mother could only add that her daughter had seemed distant and quiet, had eaten little, and had paid little attention to her husband and children for about a week but had been well before this.

Asked if her daughter had ever had convulsions, the mother said she thought she might have. About a week before, the young woman had been found semiconscious on the bathroom floor at home.

When a brain-wave recording was obtained, it showed a pattern of waves indicating grand mal and an epileptic twilight state.

The strange guises of psychomotor epilepsy

Among those who have recently been calling attention to psychomotor epilepsy as perhaps the "quintessential example of a disorder that can be mistaken for a psychiatric disturbance" is Dr. John LaWall of the University of Arizona Department of Psychiatry.

Psychomotor epilepsy, he emphasizes, can produce episodes of senseless laughter, hallucinations, outbursts of obscene language, assaultive behavior, and other abnormal behavior. In some cases, it may produce what seems to be a full-blown psychosis, with paranoia.

One of LaWall's patients was a 26-year-old man who had been rushed to an emergency room by his family physician with the brief message that the man was "psychotic and needed hospitalization." The man had smelled acetylene gas at work and, concerned about a possible explosion, had investigated and had found tanks of gas on the roof of his shop pouring into the air-conditioning system. He had called the fire and police departments, but they could find nothing wrong and suggested he see a physician.

A psychiatric consultation was requested by the emergency room staff. During the consultation, no history of behavioral problems could be elicited from the man or his wife. He denied drug use, and a mental status examination produced no evidence of delusions or hallucinations. The patient was puzzled about what had happened.

But careful further questioning finally revealed a history of short lapses of consciousness, one of which had resulted in a serious car accident. And the questioning also disclosed that the patient had once been in a building during a gas explosion.

Psychomotor epilepsy was suspected and, sure enough, an EEG revealed a brain-wave pattern indicative of such epilepsy.

"This type of case," Dr. LaWall notes, "presents the greatest diagnostic problem. There is already a psychiatric label, and the symptoms are consistent with a psychiatric disorder. However, the isolation of the symptoms in time, the bewilderment of the patient and his spouse, and the negative history are inconsistent with most psychiatric disorders. The fact from the history that led to a strong suspicion of a seizure disorder was the patient's lapses of consciousness. Thus, we should search for alterations in consciousness in the history in many psychiatric cases."

Another of LaWall's patients was an 18-year-old girl referred for admission to the psychiatric service because of a history of violent outbursts. She indicated that at times she was overcome by a feeling of rage, with or without provocation, and she would become violent, usually destroying property and occasionally attacking people. After these episodes, which lasted only minutes, she felt drained, remorseful, and confused.

Careful study revealed that she was a somewhat depressed young woman with a long-standing history of conflict with her parents. Her mother had been in a psychiatric hospital for several months when the patient was 5 years old.

Neurological tests were carried out. Both a brain scan and special brain artery X-ray studies revealed nothing abnormal. There was just a hint of abnormality in the EEG and the neurological consultants were reluctant to diagnose epilepsy.

Nevertheless, a trial of treatment with an anticonvulsant drug (diphenylhydantoin) was undertaken. And the drug worked, producing complete freedom from the seizures.

This case, Dr. LaWall points out, illustrates the difficulty in defining epilepsy. While the patient did not have a typical psychomotor seizure, she did have paroxysmal outbursts of abnormal behavior with an EEG that suggested a seizure disorder. This kind of clinical picture, in fact, which has been given the name "episodic dyscontrol," has been studied by other investigators recently, and the same anticonvulsant agent, diphenylhydantoin, has been found valuable in controlling the outbursts.

"Thus," says LaWall, "even in the face of some ambiguity, clinical suspicion should lead to consideration of a seizure disorder."

Such clinical suspicion, if it had been applied early, could have avoided thirty psychiatric hospitalizations for a young man whose psychomotor epilepsy remained undiagnosed for five years, during which time he was considered to be schizophrenic.

The misdiagnosis was uncovered by Dr. Victor R. Adebimpe of the University of Pittsburgh Department of Psychiatry and the Western Psychiatric Institute and Clinic (WPIC) in Pittsburgh.

"It is not surprising that the diagnosis of schizophrenia readily came to mind," says Adebimpe. The young man exhibited, among other things, hallucinations, ambivalence, decreased organization of thought processes, agitation, and depressive delusions at various stages. In addition, his older brother was known to be under treatment for schizophrenia.

The patient had been seen periodically in the Institute's emergency room with basically the same symptoms—frenzied movements and abnormal behavior that included muttering, grunting, humming, rolling, rocking, and crawling. Among his mutterings were the words "Hare Krishna, Hare Krishna." After three hours and two doses of the antimanic drug chlorpromazine, he would invariably emerge from an episode, rub his eyes, and calmly ask for a cigarette.

His condition had been diagnosed by various psychiatric residents as well as senior physicians as acute schizophrenia, chronic schizophrenia, acute and chronic schizophrenia, chronic schizophrenia with acute exacerbation, chronic undifferentiated schizophrenia, paranoid schizophrenia, paranoid reaction, psychotic reaction, and obsessive-compulsive personality. Most recently, a staff psychiatrist who witnessed another of his episodes had described him as showing "hypomania in the context of chronic schizo-affective illness."

He had been treated with numerous drugs used in treating psychiatric illness: chlorpromazine, trifluoperazine hydrochloride, haloperidol, fluphenazine decanoate, and lithium carbonate, either singly or in various combinations.

The uselessness of these drugs was clearly shown by the pattern of readmissions: once in 1971, five times in 1972, court commitment to a state hospital for nine months from 1972 to 1973 and one readmission to WPIC in 1973, seven in 1974, ten in 1975, and five in the first three months of 1976. At the time of the last admission the police had become tired of bringing him to the emergency room and urged his mother to consider signing commitment papers for long-term care in a state hospital.

Coming upon the man's record of previous incidents, Adebimpe became suspicious and admitted the patient to the inpatient service for study. Despite similarities to schizophrenia, the doctor noted a number of important differences. For one thing, the man's attacks had become predictable at a frequency unusual in schizophrenia. For another, schizophrenic episodes rarely last less than twenty-four hours and end spontaneously. Finally, even the abnormal activities of a schizophrenic appear to be directed at some purpose in contrast to the man's nonpurposive movements.

After observing the man while he was an inpatient, Adebimpe quickly concluded that he was not mentally ill but was suffering from psychomotor epilepsy. He was placed on antiseizure drugs and very promptly his attacks stopped.

The number of people with undiagnosed epilepsy of one kind or another who may be suffering needlessly from what seem to be mental and emotional disturbances is, of course, unknown. The number may be large or small. But even if small, the toll can be tragic enough, and all the more so since it is needless.

As Dr. LaWall points out, the range of disturbances in behavior, thought, and mood that may be seen as symptoms of epilepsy is wide, although such disturbances are usually associated with psychiatric disorders. Such symptoms may be the presenting complaints in undiagnosed cases of epilepsy. And in order to ensure accurate diagnosis, physicians should maintain a high degree of suspicion of this possibility.

Especially good reasons for suspicion, for physicians and possibly even for some patients or their families, are periodicity of symptoms, their tendency to recur at more or less regular intervals, and any alterations of consciousness, even the briefest lapses.

11. Cerebral Allergy

Among the patients seen by Dr. M. Brent Campbell, a neurologist who is Chief of Staff of Vista Hill Hospital, San Diego, was a middle-aged woman who for many years had experienced periods of unexplained depression. In the past year, severe weakness had developed and for five months, because of insomnia, appetite loss, nausea, and abdominal pain, she had been unable to do any housework. When she was found to be allergic to specific foods—pork, chocolate, milk, coffee, and peanut butter—their elimination relieved all her symptoms.

Another patient was a woman who at age 28 had begun to have episodes of confusion, headaches, chills, and vertigo that lasted twelve hours and continued at four-to-six-week intervals for eleven years. At age 32, she had suffered a convulsion and was placed on anticonvulsant medication. From age 32 to age 39, there had been recurring episodes of unexplained crying. Finally, by trial, banana, milk, chocolate, tomato, avocado, and her favorite wine were found to be the cause of her problems. Anticonvulsant medication was discontinued. On a diet free of the foods to which she was sensitive, she has had no recurrence of convulsions or other symptoms.

A 25-year-old woman is representative of many patients

seen by a Norwalk, Connecticut, allergist, Dr. Marshall Mandell. For four years she had experienced a complex of physical and mental symptoms, including extreme fatigue, tension, anxiety, fainting spells, daily periods when her vision would fail and the world about her seemed to go black. Many physicians had been unable to make a definitive diagnosis or help her. She had spent eighteen months being treated by a clinical psychologist for "emotional immaturity." Mandell's allergy tests indicated that wheat, corn, and rye led to visual blurring; house dust and some common molds produced the other disturbances. Now, avoiding the substances, she is free of symptoms.

Can allergy affect the mind? Can allergic brain and nervous system reactions be responsible in some cases for disturbances that otherwise might be considered neurotic or even psychotic?

So believes a small but zealous corps of physicians, mostly psychiatrists and allergists, who have reported working successfully on an allergic basis with thousands of patients, including many with chronic or long-standing complaints that had failed to yield to conventional treatment.

Although viewed skeptically by many if not most physicians, the concept of brain and nervous system allergic reactions is not new.

Fifty years ago, Dr. Albert Rowe, a California allergist, reported that allergy could take not only an immediate, acute physical form such as hives; it could also be chronic in nature and capable of producing mental disturbances.

In the 1920's, a number of suggestive studies pointed to the possibility. In 1921, one investigator reported in the *British Medical Journal* on two hundred cases of epilepsy with a significant number of gastrointestinal manifestations and felt there was some evidence of allergy in some of these patients.

Soon afterward, other investigators reported significant family histories of allergy in some epileptic patients. In 1923, one group studying 122 epileptic patients found 48 with positive skin tests implying allergic sensitivities. In

1927, two investigators performed skin tests for allergy on a large series of mental patients as well as epileptics. They found positive sensitivities to protein in 57 percent of the epileptic group and 37 percent of the mental group.

It was Dr. Herbert Rinkel, himself an allergy victim, who took one important step in helping in the task of trying to recognize central nervous system allergy. Rinkel reported that if suspect foods were omitted from the diet for five days or more, then the production of symptoms would be dramatic when any that were culprits were reintroduced.

Many years later, Dr. Theron Randolph at Northwestern University went a step further. He introduced the concept of a four-day fast as a means of preparing, or detoxifying, someone with a possible hidden cerebral allergy. During the fast, symptoms disappear, and when offending foods are then reintroduced, they can be associated, clearly, with the production of symptoms.

Dr. Randolph now has a special twenty-one-bed unit at Zion Benton Hospital near Chicago. There, his patients fast for at least four days, after which they receive test meals containing only a single food. After several weeks, the tests usually provide clear indications, he reports, of what foods are responsible for symptoms and need to be avoided.

But cerebral allergy may be caused by substances other than foods. Randolph has found that in some cases household pets may play a role in cerebral allergy as they do sometimes in other forms of allergy. So, too, various materials used in the home: cleaning solutions, insecticides, even gas used for cooking or heating.

The allergic phenomenon

Why should common foods or other common substances be capable of producing cerebral allergy?

Well-recognized allergic ailments, of course, are common. Hay fever, asthma, hives, skin rashes, and other sensitivity reactions—to inhalants, foods, pets, cosmetics, medicines, industrial substances—rank as the No. 1 cause of chronic discomfort, affecting an estimated thirty-one million American victims.

Allergy means "altered reaction." A person with allergy has become sensitive to a specific substance(s) harmless to the nonallergenic population. The word "specific" is important; an allergic individual may have a violent attack of asthma, for instance, when exposed to cat dander but may be comfortable with dogs and other pets.

The offending substance is called an allergen and is either protein in nature or has the capacity to combine with protein in the body. A person may be sensitive to proteins such as those in egg or milk or lobster but have no difficulty with, say, fats, such as butter, or with starches. When allergy develops to a nonprotein substance such as iodine, for example, it is believed that the offending substance itself is only a partial allergen, becoming complete when taken into the body where it combines with a protein.

In the allergic, specific allergens seem to be regarded by the body as aliens—potential threats, much as are disease organisms—and the body produces antibodies to combat the allergens just as it produces them to fend off the organisms. Allergens and antibodies interact and, in doing so, trigger the release of a chemical, histamine, which accounts for swelling and other local tissue changes. Thus, the drugs called antihistamines work in some allergies, at least to some extent, by neutralizing the histamine.

Allergens affect their body "target organs" in different ways. Airborne allergens strike the nose and air passages; food allergens are absorbed and distributed to various parts of the body, often showing their effects on the skin; contact allergens affect skin, lips, eyes; allergenic medicines may also affect the skin. Some people have physical allergies, developing hives or other allergic responses to sunlight, heat, cold, or humidity.

The symptoms of allergy depend, of course, upon the target, or shock, organ affected. If it is the nose, there may be congestion, watery discharge, and sneezing, as in hay fever; if the skin is the target, there may be rash, hives, or eczema. If the bronchial tubes are the target, asthmatic wheezing may develop.

The brain is just one more part of the body that can react to allergens.

Overlooked clues

"There are a tremendous number of chemical reactors," says Dr. Mandell, "whose illness has never previously been recognized. These people are thought to have imaginary diseases. They are treated with a shrug of the shoulder, a pat on the back, 'it's all nerves,' or 'you better go see a psychiatrist.' The truth is that they have a very definite disease."

According to Mandell, patients often bring clues to physicians but physicians don't know what to do with the clues. One of his patients told him that whenever she drank bourbon she was "disconnected" from her environment, breathed rapidly, felt depressed, and was incapable of speech. Mandell tested her with corn, from which bourbon is made. "I have," he says, "a movie showing her totally incapacitated for about thirty minutes. And this because I used the clue that she gave me."

One of his worst migraine patients was a nurse who gave him what he calls "a beautiful history." The day after having just one drink, she would experience aches and pains, irritability, and severe migraine. Nobody had bothered to exploit those clues. When he tested her with all the components of her favorite drink and came to wheat, all her symptoms were reproduced.

"There are," Dr. Mandell reports, "many forms of physical and mental illness, oftentimes very severe, in which we can demonstrate a cause and effect relationship between substances in the environment and the appearance of illness. We can actually duplicate diseases. We have turned mental illness on and off and physical illness on and off. We have had people incapacitated with acute muscular weakness and with attacks of asthma due to causes that were never suspected.

"And where do we find these causes? In the environment. These diseases are extremely common and constitute perhaps fifty to eighty percent of the daily medical practice when we exclude injuries, infections, and malignancies—problems that are described as tension, emotional, psychosomatic or 'we don't know what causes it.'

"You can have all kinds of bizarre combinations of symptoms," Dr. Mandell goes on. "They are not in the textbooks, but they happen to the same patient over and over again. If a woman comes in the office and says, 'I feel tense, I get visual blurring, my nose gets blocked up, I get cramps, gas, and vaginal itching, and my ankle hurts,' the doctor throws up his hands. This is a 'kook.' I have reproduced these symptoms again and again in people. If they have a specific inability to handle something—and this is what allergy is all about—if they can't tolerate it, if they are biochemically incapable of breaking something down, they will be sick in the tissues that respond.

"There are thousands of people in mental hospitals who don't belong there, but all we know about them is the descriptions that the psychiatrist gives. They say the patient is depressed and agitated. Anybody can say that, but the cause isn't known. They speculate on the patient's past history and inter-personal relationships. They never think of the non-personal environment that has to do with air pollution, food, and water."

When he was assistant medical director of the Fuller Memorial Sanitarium in South Attleboro, Massachusetts, Dr. William H. Philpott, a psychiatrist, studied allergic sensitivity in schizophrenic patients. In one group of fifty-three, he found that 92 percent suffered psychiatric symptoms after eating certain foods. Sixty-four percent reacted to wheat, 52 percent to corn, and 50 percent to milk. Three-fourths of the patients also responded badly to cigarette smoke, and 30 percent developed symptoms when exposed to petrochemical hydrocarbons, chemicals to be found in materials ranging from oven cleaners to gas in the kitchen stove and in automobile exhaust. Philpott extended the allergy testing to a larger series of patients and has reported that "almost every schizophrenic symptom that has ever been described turned up when we tested one hundred and fifty patients. Wheat was the commonest evoker of paranoid reactions."

At the Sanitarium, Dr. Philpott, with Dr. Mandell serving as consulting allergist, treated a patient mentioned at the beginning of this book: the adolescent girl who had been hospitalized four times between ages 13 and 16 for depression and suicidal tendencies. Particularly after her last admission, she had become increasingly withdrawn, and with shock treatment ineffective in relieving her depression, she remained in the Sanitarium for three years prior to initiation of allergy study.

When tested for sensitivities, she proved to be allergic to several substances that produced unusual reactions: saccharin, which made her dizzy, nauseated, and anxious; chlorine, in concentrations even weaker than those in drinking water, which made her depressed and afraid to swallow; lamb, which caused hand sweating, confusion, and crying.

"Once these allergens were removed," Philpott and Mandell reported, "the patient regained her equilibrium and was eligible for discharge. There has been no recurrence of symptoms since she left Fuller, and she is now preparing to enter college."

Masked allergy and food addiction

Another phenomenon may be involved in cerebral allergy, some investigators believe. This is masked allergy that can lead to a food addiction.

In the masking stage, a food may produce mild symptoms. The patient may even suspect it of doing so. But when he omits the food, the omission doesn't relieve the symptoms. On the contrary, when the food is eaten in large quantities, it may then stop the symptoms.

The relief is temporary. Several hours after eating a food that may relieve headache, fatigue, or depression, for example, symptoms begin to return and the patient then eats the food again and gets relief.

This can eventually lead to addiction to the food, and absence of the food can lead to severe withdrawal symptoms.

One problem with cerebral allergy, some investigators note, is a patient's unawareness of addiction since there are no symptoms after a food is eaten, and when delayed symptoms occur, the victim may not realize that a food eaten hours earlier is at fault.

Symptoms attributed to central nervous system allergy

Many symptoms attributed to central nervous system allergy have been reported in the medical literature over the years. They range from headaches, vertigo, and pain conditions to involuntary movements and awkwardness, antisocial behavior, anxiety, depression, and other mental disturbances.

Headache: Commonly, when a headache is due to allergy, it may start in the back part of the head and neck and spread forward over the head. It can begin gradually or suddenly, and in contrast to some other headaches, an allergic one may continue for many days or weeks.

Vertigo: There can be many reasons for vertigo which have nothing to do with allergy, but an otherwise unexplained chronic vertigo problem may be allergic. The episodes may be intermittent or may cluster, lasting three to six weeks, and may alternate with headaches. Ear noises may occur.

Sensations of imbalance: Sensations of imbalance and sometimes episodes of falling to one side or the other, when not the result of ear or other disease, may stem from allergy. The attacks may cluster, last for weeks or months, disappear, then reappear at some future time.

Sleep problems: An allergic child may have difficulty waking in the morning and may fall asleep in school. An allergic adult is likely to experience insomnia.

Muscle weakness: When muscle weakness occurs in an allergic person, it is usually accompanied by fatigue and is not relieved by sleep.

Pain: Pain may take the form of neuralgia, and when it does, it may affect neck, head, chest, abdomen, legs, or, more commonly, arms and shoulders. Or the pain may be muscular, most commonly affecting neck, shoulder, arm, and upper-back area.

Seizure-like symptoms: Somewhat resembling epilepsy in the sense that they are accompanied by a brief period of alteration of consciousness, these symptoms can include episodes of great weakness, migratory pain or paralysis, vision disturbance, confusion, garbled speech, or stuttering or stammering.

Involuntary movements: In some cases, there may be drumming of the fingers or repetitive finger movements, somewhat reminiscent of scale practice on a piano. Sudden involuntary jerking movements of head, neck, or arms and legs may occur.

Hot, cold, or shaky: Sensations of being hot and being cold and episodes of shakiness are reported to be quite common among the allergic.

Emotional immaturity: Impulsive, erratic behavior and explosive outbursts may occur. In children and teenagers, there may be stubbornness, pouting, procrastination, and aggressiveness.

Antisocial behavior: Uncooperativeness, lack of consideration for others, and loss of behavior control may occur.

Anxiety: A typical pattern of anxiety, like that of psychoneurotic anxiety, with fear and worry, may occur as the result of allergy.

Depression: Loss of appetite, loss of interest, and difficulty in concentration may occur, usually accompanied in an allergic person by weakness and fatigue. Although the depression can be severe, rarely in an allergic individual are there thoughts of suicide.

Mental dullness and slowness: These, of course, can have other causes but have been reported by several investigators as occurring sometimes with allergy.

Schizophrenia-like reactions: In the allergic, these may include changes in personal and work habits, flights of ideas, bizarre behavior, delusions, and hallucinations.

Detecting your food allergens

Anything as drastic as a four-day fast should be employed only under the supervision of a medical expert.

Are there other methods?

Dr. Frederic Speer of the Speer Allergy Clinic, Shawnee Mission, Kansas, writing not long ago in the *American Family Physician,* the publication of the American Academy of Family Physicians, reported that in his experience the chief offenders among foods responsible for various allergic manifestations, including those that may seem "neurotic," are: cow's milk, chocolate, cola, corn, eggs, the pea family (chiefly peanut, which is not a nut), citrus fruits, tomatoes, wheat and other small grains, cinnamon, and artificial food colors.

To find out which food or foods may be responsible in an individual case, Dr. Speer recommends "elimination and challenge." If two or more foods are suspect, they are removed from the diet for three weeks. Then, one is returned to the diet; later, at two-day intervals, the others are reintroduced. If only one food is suspect, it is similarly removed for three weeks. If symptoms improve with a suspected food out of the diet, then reappear when the food is added, the blame is clear.

The escalation method of detection

The escalation method of food allergy diagnosis starts with a basic hypoallergenic diet containing foods least likely to produce allergic reactions and then adds one food at a time, seeking to find the food or foods that cause trouble.

In the procedure used by Dr. M. Brent Campbell, for example, the basic diet, which is continued for at least ten days before any foods are added, consists of:

BREAKFAST:
- Pineapple juice, apple, pear, peach, prune, grape, apricot
- Tea
- Cane sugar
- Rice, cream of wheat
- Bread and butter or corn-free margarine (Coldbrook, Sunnybrook, Empress, Good Luck, Blue Bonnet)
- Evaporated milk

DINNER:
- Lamb, veal, beef
- Carrots, beets, celery, lettuce, asparagus, broccoli, squash, rutabaga, turnip, parsnip, spinach
- Oil-and-vinegar salad dressing
- Soup, using only allowable ingredients included in the rest of the diet
- White or sweet potato
- Tea
- Bread and butter or corn-free margarine
- Baked apple, pineapple, pear, peach, prune, grape, or apricot
- Evaporated milk

SUPPER:
- Pineapple, apple, peach, pear, prune, grape, or apricot
- Tea
- Carrots, beets, celery, lettuce, asparagus, broccoli, squash, rutabaga, turnip, parsnip, spinach
- Bread and butter or corn-free margarine
- Lamb, veal, beef
- Evaporated milk

Salt is allowed, as is cooking with butter or shortening, and a food eaten at one meal can be eaten at any other. Flash-frozen or water-packed vegetables (Birds Eye, Green Giant) may be used. Fruits or fruit juices must be unsweetened or water-packed. And any food wrapped in soft plastic must be removed from the wrapping for at least three days before use.

The diet is not a perfect hypoallergenic one. It may contain some foods that may be allergenic in an individual case. But in Campbell's experience, it is practical, useful in most cases.

Campbell instructs patients that they must keep a careful diary throughout, noting all foods eaten and any symptoms.

After the minimum ten days on the basic diet, foods are added one at a time. Each added food is eaten twice a day for a four-day period. If symptoms appear, the food is discontinued and four days are allowed to elapse before proceeding to the next food.

Certain foods are cross-reactive, which means that they share in common some components that may provoke allergic reactions. Most likely to be cross-reactive are members of the same food family, such as oranges and grapefruit, peas and lima beans, chocolate and cola, various nuts, and various spices. Such foods of the same family can be tried together during a food trial.

Dr. Campbell lists the following common food families that may produce allergy:

Fowl: Chicken, turkey, eggs, duck, goose
Crustaceans: Crab, crayfish, lobster, shrimp
Mammals: Beef, veal, goat, pork, rabbit, milk and milk products
Mollusks: Abalone, clam, mussel, oyster, squid
Fish: All vertebrates—bass, cod, flounder, halibut, perch, tuna, swordfish
Banana: Banana, plantain
Cashew: Cashew, mango, pistachio
Cereal: Bamboo shoots, barley, cane, corn, oats, rice, sorghum, wheat

Citrus: Orange, grapefruit, kumquat, lemon, lime, tangerine, citron
Fungi: Mushroom, yeast, truffle
Ginger: Cardamom, ginger, turmeric
Gourd: Cantaloupe, melon, pumpkin, cucumber, squash, watermelon
Laurel: Avocado, bay leaf, cinnamon, sassafras
Legume: Black-eyed pea, carob, gum acacia, gum tragacanth, licorice, lima beans, navy bean, pea, soybean, tonka bean, peanut
Lily: Garlic, onion, asparagus
Madder: Coffee
Mint: Horehound, marjoram, mint, peppermint, sage, savory, spearmint, thyme
Myrtle: Allspice, clove, guava, pimiento
Nutmeg: Mace, nutmeg
Parsley: Anise, caraway, coriander, cumin, dill, parsley, parsnip, water celery
Pepper: Black pepper, white pepper
Potato: Chili, eggplant, green pepper, potato, red pepper, tobacco, tomato
Stercuila: Cocoa, chocolate, cola beans
Walnut: Walnut, butternut, pecan, hickory nut

In the experience of Dr. Campbell, the most common food allergens, in order, have been chocolate, milk, tomato, pork, nuts, coffee, orange, corn, spices, shellfish, egg, peas, beans, alcohol, and banana.

A synthetic food to help in sensitivity testing

Recently, a synthetic food that is often used to provide complete nutrition for burn and surgical patients has been reported to be valuable in speeding and simplifying the diagnosis of food sensitivities by allergists.

Called Vivonex, it contains no proteins but instead incorporates the amino acids, or building blocks of proteins, which are needed by the body. It also incorporates all known nutrient requirements. The material is mixed with water and a desired flavor can be added, after which it may be taken chilled over cracked ice. Vivonex is meant for use only under a physician's supervision.

At the University of Southern California, Dr. Everett Hughes and other investigators studied the potential of the synthetic food in twenty-seven patients seriously ill with between eight and nineteen symptoms that could have been due to food or other allergies. Fatigue, headache, and gastrointestinal symptoms were present in more than 50 percent of the group.

Not all turned out to have food sensitivities; some had inhalant allergies. But in the twelve having predominantly food-caused trouble, a seven- to fourteen-day diet of the synthetic food eliminated symptoms. Thereafter, while continuing to use the synthetic food in part, patients added foods and could determine those they could eat and those they could not.

According to a report by Dr. Hughes in *Modern Medicine*, "The rapidity of symptom remission, the simplicity of the regimen, and the clarity of the results suggest that this procedure is of significant clinical value in the diagnosis and management of food sensitivities."

12. A Matter of Blood Sugar Plunge?

In any hierarchy of controversial disorders, hypoglycemia—low blood sugar—would certainly have to be ranked at or near the top.

That a low level of sugar in the blood can produce a remarkable variety of disturbances—mental, behavioral, and physical—is not in question. But how often?

Hypoglycemia has had a tremendous press. Vast numbers of newspaper and magazine articles and a flock of paperback books have been devoted to it.

In the view of many physicians, a cult has developed; far too much is blamed on low blood sugar levels, and while hypoglycemia does exist, it is far from common.

In the view of other physicians, however, hypoglycemia is remarkably common. Some suggest that, for one thing, "the sugar-laden American diet has led to a national epidemic of hypoglycemia." Some estimate that almost 10 percent of the population is hypoglycemic.

Because of its effects on the brain, nervous system, and adrenal glands as well, hypoglycemia can produce feelings of fatigue and weakness, dizzy spells, exhaustion, irritability, and confusion, to name only a few.

It has been credited, too, by some as being responsible

for many criminal acts. There have been representations that Adolf Hitler had a low blood sugar condition.

In Cuyahoga Falls, Ohio, when a criminal offender is referred to Probation Officer Barbara Reed, who is convinced that there are biochemical explanations for some crimes, she requires a test for hypoglycemia. If the test is positive for the condition, the two municipal judges in the community of 50,000 can order the offender to change diets, replacing sweets and starches with high protein foods, fresh vegetables and fruits, and vitamin supplements. If the offender refuses, probation can be revoked.

Mrs. Reed has reported that in one recent year her tests for hypoglycemia on 106 persons revealed that 82 percent suffered from at least fifteen symptoms of low blood sugar and that the change to a nutritional diet resulted in a "definite change in attitude and appearance" in almost all of her subjects.

One of them, a 20-year-old man arrested for criminal damage, destruction of property, and discharging a firearm, was placed on a diet after testing for hypoglycemia and studies that indicated he was paranoid and depressed and had "a deep lack of self-worth." As a result of the diet, Mrs. Reed says, the man's depression vanished and he became "optimistic, cooperative and realistic." Within four months, according to her report, he was working at a job paying $7 an hour, three months later was promoted, and his probation was lifted after ten months.

Dr. Saleem Shah, chief of the Center for Crime and Delinquency Studies at the National Institute of Mental Health, isn't convinced that hypoglycemia is commonly involved in crime but decries a lack of careful studies.

"While we are unable to estimate the degree to which hypoglycemic disorders may involve persons in trouble with the law, the base rates would probably be rather low," Shah says. "Interestingly, those rates have never been systematically measured."

Glucose and the body

Glucose, or blood sugar, is vitally important in the body economy, a source of ready energy for all tissues. It is particularly important to the brain, which is totally dependent on glucose for its energy needs.

You absorb dietary carbohydrates—sugars and starches—after they are first broken down into simple sugars—glucose, fructose, and galactose. The glucose is what counts: galactose and fructose are changed by the liver into glucose.

Soon after a meal, the blood sugar (glucose) level goes up and each 100 milliliters of blood may contain as much as 130 to 140 milligrams of glucose. In about two hours, the glucose level drops off to a level of 60 to 90. And it stays this way between meals.

The liver helps to keep the level constant. When carbohydrates are consumed and absorbed as glucose, any excess of glucose beyond what is immediately needed in the blood is stored in the liver as glycogen. As body tissues utilize glucose and thus reduce its level in the blood, glycogen is quickly converted back to glucose and released by the liver into the blood circulation. The kidneys also help in glucose level control by taking any marked excess of glucose (usually anything more than 170 to 180 milligrams per 100 milliliters) out of the blood and excreting it in the urine.

The pancreas, of course, is very much a factor in blood glucose control through its secretion of the hormone insulin. It is insulin that ushers glucose from the blood into tissue cells and stimulates its use by the cells. Insulin also acts on the liver to convert excess glucose to glycogen. Other hormones as well, from the pituitary and adrenal glands, play a role in blood glucose control.

With a disturbance of glucose regulatory processes, there can be hyperglycemia, or diabetes, with its excess of sugar in the blood, or, on the other hand, hypoglycemia, with its abnormally low levels.

Hypoglycemic symptoms

Blood sugar levels of about 40 milligrams per 100 milliliters or below begin to cause symptoms. The symptoms can vary considerably both in type and degree. Generally, the more rapid the fall in blood sugar, the more prominent are the symptoms. It is even possible, authorities report, that if blood sugar level goes down very gradually it can reach values of as little as 5 to 10 milligrams without any symptoms.

When symptoms do occur, commonly the initial ones may include headache, faintness, confusion, restlessness, clouded consciousness, hunger, irritability, and visual disturbances.

Other symptoms may occur when the adrenal glands, in response to the falling blood sugar level, secrete the hormone epinephrine. These may include anxiety, tremor, perspiration, racing heartbeat, pallor, and tingling of the fingers and around the mouth.

Spontaneous hypoglycemia

There are two types of low blood sugar conditions, spontaneous and reactive.

Spontaneous hypoglycemia, which is less common, occurs in the fasting state. It can sometimes, but rarely, result from inability of normal production of glucose to keep up with excessive glucose use, as in vigorous exercise or pregnancy. Sometimes the problem may lie with failure of glucose production due to extensive liver disease.

Spontaneous hypoglycemia also can result from excessive use of glucose through insulin overproduction by an insulin-secreting tumor of the islet cells of the pancreas which normally are responsible for insulin production. While such tumors are uncommon, as many as 90 percent of them are surgically curable.

Occasionally, excessive glucose utilization may be due to

a deficiency of a pituitary, adrenal, or thyroid gland hormone important in having an opposing effect to insulin. With such deficiency, there is an excessive insulin effect and, as a consequence, abnormally high use of glucose.

Reactive hypoglycemia

Reactive hypoglycemia, the most common type of low blood sugar, is characterized by the appearance of symptoms within two to four hours after eating.

It can follow, but doesn't always, after stomach surgery in which some of the stomach is removed because of peptic ulcer or other reason. Glucose then may be absorbed with abnormal rapidity into the blood circulation, and there may then be a subsequent outpouring of an excess of insulin so the glucose level falls rapidly.

Reactive hypoglycemia may be due to mild diabetes and sometimes may be the first indication of it. In such cases, there is a delayed insulin response after a meal, particularly one heavy in carbohydrates. Soon after a meal, blood sugar level is very high. The very high level then causes insulin to be secreted in excess by the pancreas, with consequent sudden, rapid lowering of blood sugar levels.

Reactive hypoglycemia also can occur in some cases in response to use of alcohol or other drugs such as salicylates (aspirin and aspirinlike compounds), aminobenzoic acid, haloperidol, propoxyphene, and chlorpromazine.

Another type of reactive hypoglycemia that follows a carbohydrate-rich meal is known as "functional" and its mechanism is unknown.

Diagnosing the problem

The symptoms of hypoglycemia are not unique to low blood sugar conditions. They are like those of many other possible disorders.

So an essential for diagnosis of hypoglycemia is a finding of low blood sugar associated with the symptoms. Some physicians believe that hypoglycemia should be documented by at least two blood glucose tests when a patient is having symptoms, although getting blood specimens during transient episodes can be difficult in some cases.

When the symptoms occur—within four hours after a meal or after a fast, either overnight or more prolonged—is an important consideration in determining suitable diagnostic tests. In fasting hypoglycemia, it is important to do tests to make certain whether an islet cell tumor, which may be surgically correctable, is present.

Also, in fasting hypoglycemia, other possible physical causes may need to be considered, including liver disease that requires treatment and deficiencies of pituitary, adrenal, or thyroid hormones that can be overcome.

For reactive hypoglycemia, a glucose tolerance test often is a valuable diagnostic aid. The usual test consists of giving the subject about 100 grams of pure glucose in a drink in the morning without other food for breakfast. Blood samples are then collected periodically for at least three and often five hours, and the glucose present in all blood samples is plotted on a graph to display the changes in blood sugar levels. The pattern on the graph usually distinguishes between the common types of reactive hypoglycemia—those caused by stomach surgery, mild diabetes, and the functional type.

When the problem is the result of surgery, it can often be managed well with a drug such as propantheline (Pro-Banthine), which works to slow carbohydrate absorption and to dampen insulin secretion.

When the fault lies with mild diabetes, weight reduction sometimes is enough to correct it. If not, antidiabetic medication may be used.

When reactive hypoglycemia is functional—without organic cause—a diet high in protein and low in carbohydrate taken at frequent intervals in small servings is usually effective.

The sugar connection

If some investigators are right, functional reactive hypoglycemia is common today, affecting to some degree almost one of every ten people, because of both what we eat and the way we eat.

The "what" revolves about the consumption of a lot of carbohydrates and, in particular, an excess of sugar. When sugar or starch is in a meal, it tends to be absorbed quickly and gets into the blood quickly as glucose. If protein or fat is in a meal, its digestion products also will be converted in part into glucose but more slowly.

Quite normally, when blood glucose rises, the rise is only temporary since the glucose elevation stimulates the pancreas to secrete insulin, which leads to the storage of excess glucose in the liver as glycogen, with the blood level falling back toward normal.

But if large quantities of sugar are consumed, especially between meals when no other food constituents are in the intestinal tract that might possibly delay absorption, trouble can develop.

There is then, maintains Professor John Yudkin, Britain's well-known physician and nutritionist, a rapid rise of blood glucose, and an excessive amount of insulin is secreted in response to the sharp rise. Because of this, the subsequent fall of blood glucose is excessive. The level becomes abnormally low, and if it becomes low enough, symptoms of hypoglycemia appear.

There is some evidence, too, according to Dr. Yudkin, that continued high intake of sugar can, at least for a time, result in an increased sensitivity of the pancreas, so that it responds more readily still by an increased secretion of insulin, and hypoglycemia becomes even more likely.

"How then do you treat hypoglycemia? Well, if you don't bother to think out the consequences of what I have just said," Yudkin observes, "then clearly you treat a person with low blood sugar by giving sugar. And the effect is pretty miraculous: within a few minutes, all the sweating and weakness and dizziness disappear. But now think back for a moment and you will see that this, however effective, is in the long run just what should not be done.

"What you need do is to prevent the large swing in blood glucose that each time ends in an excessive fall. Only foods that result in a gentle rise in blood sugar should be eaten, so that an excessive output of insulin by the pancreas is not evoked. That is why the best treatment for a lack of sugar in the blood is the paradoxical treatment of avoiding sugar in your diet as much as possible."

Drs. E. Cheraskin and W. M. Ringsdorf, Jr., of the University of Alabama in Birmingham also point the finger of blame at sugar. They note that hypoglycemia, which may be induced by sugar, may trigger a craving for sweets along with such a crazy-quilt pattern of physical and mental complaints as to be easy to pass off as "just an attack of nerves."

Most hypoglycemics, they charge, are regarded as "cranks" or "complainers" by their families, "hypochondriacs" by their doctors, and "neurotics" by society. And milder cases may be advised: "You'll get over it—eat something sweet when the craving hits." This, they note, much as does Yudkin, is the worst thing a hypoglycemic can do, "for the more sweets eaten, the more insulin is released, the lower the blood sugar levels plunge, the more sugar is craved . . . on and on in a never-ending cycle."

Cheraskin and Ringsdorf believe that every tenth person inherits a pancreas that is especially sensitive to and incapable of handling large intakes of sugar, overproducing insulin quite easily as a result.

If so, the American diet—and, for that matter, the diet of much of the so-called "civilized" world—amounts to a steady insult to the sensitive pancreases.

For centuries, sucrose—the technical name for sugar from cane or beets—was sold only by apothecaries, who measured out the granules by the ounce. Only the rich could afford it, and even they could not splurge since the supply was short. In Elizabethan times, the total consumption for all of England amounted to only about 88 tons a year.

It was less than a century ago, when Latin America went in for sugar cane cultivation and Europeans worked out a process for refining sugar beets, that production of table sugar began to soar. In 1850, total world production was only 3.5 million tons; by 1950, it was 35 million; currently, it exceeds 70 million.

And in the United States and Western industrialized nations, the per capita consumption of sugar is up to 140 to 150 pounds a year, more than 2 pounds a week. Commonly now, a startlingly large proportion of daily calories, upward of 500, comes from sugar. Of the 525 pounds of food consumed per person per year in the United States on a dry basis, sucrose makes up one-fifth.

Sources of sugar intake are not by any means always obvious. Even people conscious of weight and the need for dieting, those who dutifully say no to pies and cakes and don't use sugar in their coffee or tea, get plenty of hidden sugar.

Sugar is to be found in the seemingly most unlikely products: in ketchup, relish, canned soups, frozen pizza, bottled salad dressings. Sugar is put into many prepared "convenience" foods. A chart prepared by the Center for Science in the Public Interest showed the sugar content of some sixty-five fabricated foods. Some contained as much as 68 percent sugar. Even many common medications, prescription and over-the-counter, contain sugar.

How we eat may also be a factor in hypoglycemia.

Many skip breakfast entirely. Many others take little if anything more than coffee and a sweet roll, after which blood sugar levels rise but then within two or three hours dip down. Temporarily, coffee and another sweet roll or its equivalent at about ten in the morning make the victim feel better.

"If," say Drs. Cheraskin and Ringsdorf, "by lunchtime his nerves demand a quick drink or he skips that meal and satisfies his hunger with more coffee, a sweet soft drink, or a heavily refined carbohydrate repast [which also is turned to glucose and rapidly absorbed, with an effect on insulin secretion similar to that of sucrose], he will be tense, nervous, and irritable by two, in worse shape by four, and even a well-balanced dinner will not restore his physical and mental equilibrium. He is exhausted, yet he may get only a few hours' sleep each night."

After an overnight fast, the body needs a good nutritional start in the morning. Something in the neighborhood of 15 to 20 grams of high-quality protein are needed to sustain blood sugar levels during the morning.

As we noted at the beginning of this chapter, hypoglycemia ranks high among controversial disorders. And that is especially so for the reactive type.

At its 1977 annual session in Dallas, the American College of Physicians held a special panel discussion on "the hypoglycemic dilemma." Members of the panel agreed that reactive hypoglycemia is highly controversial and overdiagnosed but that other hypoglycemic states often may go unrecognized.

According to panel moderator Dr. Marvin D. Saperstein, University of California, San Francisco, School of Medicine, any discussion of reactive hypoglycemia will create vehement arguments over whether such a disease even exists. Dr. Thomas J. Merimee, University of Florida College of Medicine, Gainesville, expressed the conviction that reactive hypoglycemia "may be a psychosomatic manifestation in individuals who have acute anxiety that has been transferred into somatic symptoms following meals."

Other panelists felt it unwise to disregard a patient's complaints but to reassure him that if he has the symptoms, he will not be harmed. But Dr. Arthur H. Rubenstein, University of Chicago Pritzker School of Medicine, was more positive: a diet stressing high protein and low concentrated carbohydrates, he reported, can often significantly help symptomatic patients.

13. When the "Nervous" Stomach Isn't

Among the most common of all disorders are those affecting the gut. One-half the population of the United States complains about something wrong with the digestive system. Sixty percent of adult patients who seek help from primary physicians do so because of a g-i problem. We spend more than $218 million a year for laxatives, $127 million for antacids, and even more for calmatives, antispasmodics, and so on.

Can emotions affect the gut? Of course. For centuries it has been observed that fear can produce a dry mouth and an empty sensation at the pit of the stomach.

Back in 1822, when a shotgun blast tore off the skin and muscles of the upper part of the abdomen of Alexis St. Martin and, in addition, the outer layer of the wall of the stomach, the best that Dr. William Beaumont, a young U.S. Army surgeon, could do was to stitch the stomach edges to the skin. Happily for himself and for science, St. Martin lived with the hole in his stomach. Beaumont, with St. Martin's cooperation, could look in and see the stomach, noting changes in its appearance brought about by excitement and anger.

An even more important contribution to an understanding of the effects of emotions on the gut was made by a man named Tom. When he was a boy of nine, Tom had swallowed steaming-hot clam chowder which burned and blocked his esophagus, making it useless, requiring surgery to provide an artificial opening from outside into his stomach. Tom had learned to chew his food, then remove it from his mouth and introduce it into a funnel attached to a rubber tube leading to his stomach.

He got along until one day in New York while doing physical labor he began to bleed from the opening that apparently had been irritated by his movements at work. He was hospitalized and while in the hospital was persuaded by two investigators, Drs. Stewart Wolf and Harold Wolff, then doing research on the effects of emotions on the body, to become a subject for study.

The two researchers noted many phenomena in the course of the study. When Tom became angry or resentful, they could see the pink color of the stomach change to red and stomach juices flow freely. On the other hand, when he was sad, fearful, or depressed, the stomach lining became pale and secretions decreased.

When food was introduced while Tom was angry or anxious, it would be out of the stomach in less than usual time. When it was introduced when he was depressed, it might remain in the stomach undigested for many hours.

Since then, other investigations have established that disturbances elsewhere in the gut may be caused or accentuated by emotional disturbances. Anger, resentment, guilt, anxiety, conflict, and feelings of being in overwhelming situations have been found capable of increasing mucus and other secretions in the intestines and of increasing contractions and other activities there, producing diarrhea and other discomfort. And depression, fear, feelings of futility or defeat have been shown to decrease secretions and other activities, sometimes producing constipation.

So, clearly enough, the digestive system can react to emotional stress.

Yet, in some disorders, very common ones, which often have been considered psychogenic, recent research indicates that the fault may lie elsewhere.

The so-called irritable bowel syndrome

The irritable bowel syndrome, the most common of gastrointestinal problems, is also known by such names as spastic colon and mucous colitis, although the latter is erroneous since colitis means inflammation of the colon and the irritable, or spastic, colon is not inflamed.

It has often been considered to be a disorder of civilization, reflecting the stresses of American living. The irritable bowel syndrome can cause severe discomfort, sometimes severe enough to disrupt normal life.

The symptoms are variable and, at best, never pleasant. There may be abdominal distention and abdominal pain, sharp and knifelike or deep and dull. There may be constipation or diarrhea, or one alternating with the other. Excess mucus may appear in stools, but no blood unless hemorrhoids also happen to be present, and they commonly happen in chronically constipated people.

Many of those with the syndrome complain of lack of appetite in the morning, nausea, heartburn, or excessive belching, and there may also be complaints of weakness, palpitation, headaches, faintness, sleeping trouble.

The diagnosis of irritable bowel syndrome is made when such symptoms are present yet thorough examination of the colon and the stool shows no evidence of disease.

Emotional stress has long been regarded as a prime factor in the irritable bowel. Many physicians have found that patients with the problem often are tense, anxious, and given to emotional ups and downs. There is often a history of overwork, inadequate sleep, hurried and irregular meals, and abuse of laxatives.

Colon activities, of course, are under nervous system control. There are nerve impulses that stimulate activity; others that inhibit it; and, normally, a fine balance between the two kinds allows gastrointestinal contents to pass smoothly through the colon.

If the balance is disturbed, material may not move through normally, being either slowed down or speeded up. One function of the colon is to retrieve water from the material passing through. If the material stays around long, excess amounts of water may be retrieved, to the point where the feces become dry and hard and the victim becomes constipated. On the other hand, if the material doesn't stay around long enough, allowing little chance for water absorption, there may be diarrhea, with loose, unformed stools. And when the muscles of the colon go into spasm, as they commonly do, pain results.

Symptoms of irritable bowel syndrome are intermittent and recurrent, with individual episodes lasting sometimes for days but not uncommonly for weeks or months. And, to make matters worse, quite often, in addition to everything else, fatigue, depression, anxiety, and difficulty with mental concentration occur.

Treatment has often included efforts to reassure a patient that there is no organic problem and that it would be best to avoid stressful conditions as much as possible. Sedatives and tranquilizers often have been used, plus antispasmodic agents, the latter not infrequently at the expense of dry mouth, blurred vision, or drowsiness. Often, too, a bland diet and avoidance of raw fruits and vegetables have been recommended.

Irritable or irritated?

But is the irritable bowel syndrome aptly named? Is the colon really irritable? Some surveys have indicated that the so-called irritable bowel, or colon, is responsible for up to 60 percent of patients attending gastrointestinal clinics in whom no abnormality of the colon or any other part of the digestive tract can be demonstrated. It would seem highly unlikely, on evolutionary grounds, that so many people, so high a proportion of the population, should be born with a congenitally irritable intestine.

It was an English surgeon, Neil Painter, who first took a hard new look at the irritable bowel problem just a few years ago and suggested that a better term would be "irritated" (rather than "irritable") bowel syndrome, that the bowel is not irritable but rather is being abnormally irritated, and that the irritation comes from diet—not what is in the diet but what is left out.

Painter came to this conclusion—for which substantiating evidence has since been coming from the work of others as well as his own—by way of studies of another common digestive system problem, diverticular disease, which is believed by many to be particularly prone to develop in people with "irritable" colons.

A diverticulum—from the Latin for "to turn aside"—is an outpouching, or sac, protruding outward from the intestinal lining into the intestinal wall. In diverticular disease, there may be scores, even hundreds, of diverticula, benign at the start and sometimes remaining so. But the pouches can trap feces, and about 20 percent of those with diverticula develop inflammation, or diverticulitis, which may produce pain in the lower left abdomen, nausea, vomiting, distention, chills, and fever.

Diverticula are common. A third of all Americans over 45 and two-thirds of those over 60 have them. And while medication sometimes has helped when diverticulitis has developed, often surgery has been required.

Years ago, Painter, in pioneering studies at Cambridge University, had measured colonic pressures in diverticular disease and coupled the pressure measurements with X-ray movies of the colon. He had established that the pressures were abnormally high and that they occurred as the walls of the colon had to clamp down hard in efforts to move along the small, hard stools of diverticular disease patients who commonly had long histories of constipation. It was this high-pressure clamping down that pushed hard on the lining of the colon so that eventually the lining pushed through the colon's muscular wall, forming pouches.

Years were to go by before, in 1967, Painter began a study that was to change the whole outlook for, and method of treatment of, diverticular disease.

Something else had been going on. Many British investigators, notably Denis Burkitt, a distinguished surgeon who had spent many years in Africa, and Dr. Hugh Trowell, who had also spent time as a missionary physician in Africa, had become impressed by the fact that many disorders common in highly industrialized Western nations such as Britain and the United States didn't exist in native African villages. Among those disorders were constipation and diverticular disease.

After considering many differences between African villagers and Britons and Americans, the investigators had decided that the critical one was fiber. Africans got plenty of it in the foods they ate. Westerners got very little; it had been refined out of cereal grains, where it was particularly plentiful, in the course of producing refined cereals and refined white flour.

The investigators began to carry out studies among British patients. Clearly, constipation could be relieved when constipated subjects ate whole-meal breads rather than refined white bread, or when bran, the part of the grain rich in fiber and removed in refining, was added to the diet.

Influenced by these findings, Painter set up his study with diverticular disease patients. In terms of conventional medicine, it was a daring study. The medical rule had been: For diverticular disease, always a diet low in fiber, as free as possible of roughage. The idea had been that so-called roughage would be irritating to a colon full of pouches.

But, as studies by Painter and others demonstrated, fiber is not roughage. In the intestinal tract, it absorbs water and, in so doing, gives bulk to the stool. With the bulk, there were no more of the pebbly, hard stools of constipation, but, rather, soft, easily evacuated stools.

In his study, which took in seventy patients with diverticular disease, Painter prescribed a high-fiber diet. The patients ate bran cereal, porridge, whole-meal bread, plenty of fruits and vegetables. They were also told to take two teaspoons of unprocessed bran three times a day.

Bowel habits changed dramatically. Constipation disappeared; soft motions were passed regularly and easily with no straining at stool. And with the diet change, symptoms of diverticular disease were relieved in 88.6 percent of the patients, even in those with symptoms so severe that they had been considered candidates for surgery to remove the affected portion of the colon. None required surgery.

Painter's study, soon duplicated by the studies of others, completely changed the treatment of diverticular disease.

Not long afterward, Painter took a look at the irritable bowel problem.

It seemed to him that there was double significance in the fact that a high-fiber diet could relieve the symptoms of diverticular disease, for the relief is achieved even though the diverticula, or pouches, remain. Evidently, then, the symptoms weren't due to the diverticula. Where did they stem from?

It seemed to Painter that if a fiber-deficient diet can damage the colon enough to produce diverticula, it had to be highly unlikely that the colon, and often only one region of it (the sigmoid), is the only part of the gut adversely affected by a fiber-deficient diet. The symptoms could well originate in other parts of the digestive tract that had not adapted to a low-residue diet. That could explain not only why such upper-intestinal symptoms as nausea and heartburn accompany diverticular disease but also how a high-fiber diet relieves them. And that, he believed, could also throw some light on the origin of the symptoms of irritable colon.

And, in fact, before long, Painter was able to report that irritable bowel symptoms also often respond to a high-fiber diet.

One of the first to confirm Painter's finding was Dr. Joseph L. Piepmeyer, a medical officer in the U.S. Naval Reserve stationed at the Beaufort, North Carolina, Naval Hospital. In a study with thirty patients with irritable bowel symptoms, Piepmeyer prescribed 8 to 10 teaspoons of bran a day for three weeks. Four patients dropped out because they found the bran unpalatable. But twenty-three of the twenty-six who used the bran, 88 percent, reported improvement in their symptoms.

In a scientifically controlled trial at the Bristol Royal Infirmary in England, investigators divided patients with irritable bowel syndrome into two groups, one receiving a high-fiber diet, the other, for comparison, a low-fiber diet. After six weeks on the high-fiber diet, there was substantial improvement in symptoms and a clearly measurable beneficial change in colon activity. No such improvement occurred on the low-fiber regimen. Patients with irritable bowel syndrome should be encouraged, the investigators urge, to increase their daily intake of fiber.

The very common matter of milk intolerance

Until recently, a Baltimore woman was one of a very large group of people suffering from repeated, unexplained episodes of abdominal bloating, cramps, and diarrhea. For her, as for others, no organic disease could be found.

Today, she is very happy to be free of the symptoms and also to know that her problem was no neurotic manifestation but rather a simple intolerance to milk or, more precisely, to a particular substance in milk.

The problem is widespread. Until only a decade or so ago, the intolerance was considered an uncommon digestive disorder, largely limited to rare newborns with congenital deficiencies or derangements. Now it is estimated to affect about thirty million Americans.

"Over the last ten years," reports one of the pioneer investigators, Dr. Theodore M. Bayless, associate professor of medicine at Johns Hopkins University School of Medicine and Physician to the Johns Hopkins Hospital, Baltimore, "milk intolerance has been increasingly recognized as a factor in some patients with the irritable colon syndrome, postgastrectomy [stomach operation] diarrhea, and, more commonly of all, unexplained abdominal pain and flatulence; it has also been recognized as a factor in some patients with known organic causes of diarrhea, such as ulcerative colitis or Crohn's disease."

The milk sugar

Milk contains lactose, a sugar that is indigestible. But an enzyme produced in the small intestine and called lactase acts on lactose and splits it into simple sugars that are readily absorbed. Intolerance develops in the absence of adequate amounts of the enzyme. The undigested lactose passes on through the gut, causing disturbances along the way.

And recent studies indicate that much of the capacity to produce the enzyme is lost at an early age in many people. In an infant, lactase levels rise to a peak at birth and remain high throughout infancy when milk is a major source of nutrition.

When it comes to most other mammals, it has long been recognized that lactase levels start to drop off after weaning, with the shift from milk to other sources of nourishment. But it was long assumed that man somehow is an exceptional mammal capable of maintaining high lactase levels throughout life. Now it has become evident that postweaning decline is common in man, although the degree of fall-off can vary markedly among different groups.

Recent surveys have established that in North America 58 to 100 percent of people of Eskimo, American Indian, sub-Sahara African, and Asian extraction are lactose intolerant. Among American whites, the incidence is lower but still ranges up to as high as 24 percent.

Some scientists believe that most of the world's adults cannot digest lactose, and that it is not intolerance but rather lactose tolerance that is the abnormal condition. The abnormality, they suggest, may have come about this way: Before the domestication of milk-giving animals, man, like other mammals, had high lactase levels during nursing, followed by a marked drop after weaning. With dairying, the normal state of lactose intolerance changed in some populations as "aberrant" individuals retained high intestinal lactase activity throughout life.

Based on the latest available studies, it now appears that

the approximately 30 million people in the United States who are intolerant of large amounts of lactose are made up of several groups: about 16 million white adults and teenagers of northern European extraction, 10.5 million black adults and teenagers, 2.4 million Jewish adults and teenagers, and some 800,000 children of elementary school age belonging in those groups.

And although some of these people experience symptoms only after a large intake of milk, at least half are likely to be affected by just one or two glasses.

Determining if you're intolerant

If you have symptoms of bloating, cramps, and diarrhea that might be related to lactose intolerance, how can you make certain that they are?

One way is to have a physician carry out a lactose tolerance test, which simply involves measurements on a sample of blood drawn after you have consumed a specified amount of milk. If you have no lactase deficiency and your problems have no relation to intolerance, the blood will contain high levels of sugar because the lactase supply was adequate to convert the lactose into an absorbable form, permitting it to get into the blood. Conversely, low blood levels point to intolerance.

There are other methods of detecting lactose intolerance. You can cut back on your milk intake or stop using milk entirely for a period of a week and see if symptoms disappear. Or, conversely, you can drink two glasses of cold milk, which seems to produce symptoms more often than warm milk, on an empty stomach and that may be all that is needed to demonstrate the relationship between milk and abdominal symptoms.

What can you do?

If lactose intolerance should prove to be the cause of your symptoms, there is nothing complex about avoiding the discomforts.

Most lactose-intolerant people, although not able to consume large amounts of milk with impunity, can take milk in reasonable quantity in cereal or coffee. You may also find, as do many, that you have no difficulties when you take your milk with a meal rather than by itself and when you avoid ice-cold milk.

You can also use milk alternatives. Yogurt, hard cheeses, and similar dairy products have a lower content of lactose because it has already been fermented into lactic acid during processing.

A new development also holds promise for the lactose intolerant. At several universities, researchers have worked with a lactase enzyme produced by yeast. When added to milk in small amounts, it has been effective in breaking down the lactose. Milk treated with it is identical nutritionally to regular milk. The one difference is a sweeter taste, which most users have found acceptable and some consider desirable. The enzyme-treated milk can be used for drinking as fresh skim or whole milk and for making ice cream, yogurt, cottage cheese, and puddings.

At least one dairy—in Sumter, South Carolina—has begun to pretreat milk with the enzyme and many others are expected to follow.

Meanwhile, the enzyme product, under the name of Lact-Aid, is becoming available in supermarkets and in drug and other retail stores in little packets that can be added to milk at home.

The heartburn story

Heartburn hardly needs any definition. At one point or other, most of us have experienced the burning sensation in the esophagus felt behind the breastbone.

But if an occasional experience is commonplace, there are people who suffer from chronic, frequently recurring heartburn.

Look up heartburn in popular health or medical books and chances are you will find it said that "nervous people, those under great stress" are the chronic sufferers. And even some professional texts and other books contain such statements as "there is no doubt that emotional disturbance, excitement, and nervous tension are frequent causes of heartburn."

Certainly, psychogenic influences can contribute to heartburn in many cases. But not by any means are all sufferers necessarily emotionally disturbed, excited, nervously tense, or under great stress. And even among those who are, there can be more to the story.

The heartburn reflux

Heartburn involves reflux, or abnormal return, of material, including acid, from the stomach up into the esophagus where the acidity irritates and burns. Commonly, the reflux is accompanied by spasm, or abnormal contraction, of the muscles of the esophagus. The spasm commonly leads to a third phenomenon: air swallowing, which is the body's way to try to counteract the spasm. The swallowing helps to distend the esophagus and in so doing may interrupt the muscle contraction. And, in fact, after swallowing, some of the air is belched up and the belching also helps to interrupt the spasm. Not all swallowed air, however, is burped immediately and some may remain to distend the stomach and produce a bloated feeling.

But the prime problem lies in a musclelike area, about an inch long, at the lower end of the esophagus where it joins the stomach. Called the lower esophageal sphincter (LES), the area serves as a valve. It opens to let food pass from the esophagus to the stomach. It then closes snugly to prevent regurgitation of stomach contents. Or should.

The importance of the LES has been recognized only recently. It used to be thought that chronic reflux problems resulted from a hiatal hernia, an abnormal opening in the diaphragm, the domelike muscle between abdomen and chest, through which the esophagus passes. When the opening is abnormal, it can allow part of the stomach to protrude up into the chest, and such protrusion was believed to be a common cause of stomach-content return into the esophagus. But in the last half dozen years, many investigators, among them Dr. F. Henry Ellis, Jr., of the Lahey Clinic Foundation, Boston, have been finding that not all people with hiatal hernia have heartburn and some with severe heartburn have no hiatal hernia.

The basic trouble really lies with sphincter incompetence. In the last half dozen years, too, studies by Dr. Sidney Cohen and other University of Pennsylvania, Philadelphia, investigators have established that in the normal individual, the resting, or basal, sphincter pressure is high enough (about 15 millimeters of mercury) to keep it snugly closed against reflux. The studies also reveal that the LES pressure rises when food is eaten and also in response to increases in intra-abdominal pressure, such as occur during exercise, again serving to prevent reflux.

On the other hand, the resting pressure in patients with reflux is below normal (under 10 millimeters of mercury) and the pressure fails to rise as much as in normal people after meals and during exercise. As a result of failure of the LES to close tightly enough, reflux may occur under resting conditions and during sleep as well as after eating and during exercise.

Although how sphincter incompetence develops is still unknown, the discovery of its role in chronic heartburn has been of great practical value. It has led to University of Pennsylvania and other studies that now reveal what can affect the sphincter for good or bad, what substances, including foods and drugs, reduce its pressure and act to prevent firm closing and what substances have an opposite, beneficial effect.

The influential foods

The Pennsylvania studies indicate that LES pressure is stimulated by gastrin, a hormone secreted by the stomach during eating and to a lesser extent at other times. On the other hand, another hormone, cholecystokinin, which may be released during eating, tends to reduce LES pressure. And certain foods can contribute to heartburn because of their effects on gastrin, cholecystokinin, and acid secretion as well.

Fatty foods stimulate cholecystokinin secretion and so reduce LES pressure. Sugar-rich foods can play a role in reflux because they stimulate stomach acid secretion without at the same time stimulating increased LES pressure. Protein, however, stimulates gastrin secretion and thus increases LES pressure, and tends to counteract the effects of fats and sugars. In studies at the U.S. Naval Hospital, Philadelphia, Drs. Donald O. Castell and Otto T. Nebel have found that LES pressure in normal volunteers consistently increases after a protein meal but significantly decreases after fatty meals.

Because of differing individual sensitivities, some foods encourage heartburn in some but not all victims. Among the most common offenders in this group are garlic, peppers, and onions.

Alcohol can be troublesome for some. It diminishes sphincter pressure while at the same time increasing acid secretion.

The role of coffee is questionable. It had been thought that the caffeine in coffee increases acid secretion and reduces sphincter pressure. But in special studies in Philadelphia, Dr. Cohen has found that while coffee does indeed stimulate acid secretion, it increases rather than decreases sphincter pressure.

Still some physicians, on the basis of experience with heartburn patients, believe that coffee sometimes may be a culprit. They report that heartburn incidence has declined markedly in some patients, previously heavy coffee users, who switched to decaffeinated coffee or eliminated coffee entirely. They also note benefits in some patients who cut down on cola drinks, coffee, and tea, all of which contain caffeine.

Peculiarly, citrus juices give some people heartburn although why is an enigma. There are other enigmas as well:

why deep-fried foods commonly cause trouble while pan-fried often may not; and why fresh bread, especially rye and pumpernickel, may cause problems for some yet stale bread will not.

Smoking and heartburn

Cigarette smoking has been suspect. But it remained for British investigators at the Royal Infirmary, Hull, to provide a convincing demonstration.

Working with men and women volunteers, aged 24 to 71, all chronic smokers and heartburn victims, Drs. C. Stanciu and J. R. Bennett used measuring devices to record sphincter pressures. The pressures fell by a mean of 40 percent during smoking, beginning within one to four minutes after a cigarette was lighted. The measuring instrumentation also permitted recording of any acidity in the esophagus as an indication that reflux was taking place. And refluxes did, indeed, occur and were severe enough to produce heartburn 68 percent of the time during or after smoking.

Coping with heartburn

A first step for any chronic heartburn sufferer, sometimes the only one needed, is a trial of dietary changes, reducing the intake of foods that lower sphincter pressure and increasing intake of those that raise the pressure.

That means avoiding as much as possible foods cooked in fat or rich in fats and foods high in sugar. Emphasis should be on protein-rich foods, valuable for raising sphincter pressure and for counteracting the pressure-reducing effects of unavoidable fats and sugar in foods.

Other dietary measures that could be worth a trial: reduction or elimination of coffee intake or a switch to decaffeinated, and a period of avoidance of onions, garlic, or other foods you suspect may be contributing to your heartburn.

Other obvious measures that may be worth a trial to determine the effect: reduction or elimination of drinking and smoking.

Because a recumbent position soon after a meal, while the stomach is still full, tends to make reflux easier, lying down shortly after dinner or eating soon before bedtime should be avoided. After two hours or more, there is much less chance for discomfort.

Also helpful for some people: elevating the head of the bed about 6 or 8 inches on blocks so gravitational forces can help counteract any tendency to heartburn. And because tight clothes can raise intra-abdominal pressure, they should be avoided.

Antacids? They don't have any effect on the cause of reflux, sphincter incompetence, but they do react with and neutralize acid and can provide relief.

Physicians, however, caution that the stronger the antacid activity and the more immediately effective, the more likely an acid rebound, a stimulation of the stomach to produce more acid within half an hour or so. Many people find that bicarbonate of soda, for example, is more quickly effective than commercial antacids, but the fast relief departs rapidly too. And frequent use of bicarbonate can be unwise because of its sodium content and excessive sodium intake can raise blood pressure.

Some commercial antacids contain calcium carbonate or another calcium salt. They can be suitable for occasional use, but a large intake of calcium-containing preparations over a prolonged period may lead to excess calcium in the blood and kidney disorder. Among antacids favored by many physicians are those containing no calcium but formulated with aluminum and magnesium trisilicates and hydroxides, such as Mylanta II, Maalox, and Gelusil.

For 80 percent or more of chronic heartburn victims, dietary changes, avoidance of recumbency soon after meals, and perhaps occasional use of an antacid can provide satisfactory relief. If you need to take an antacid more than once or twice a week, it's advisable to get medical help to make certain that serious disease, such as peptic ulcer, malignancy, or heart trouble, is not involved and that, in fact, reflux is causing the discomfort.

One effective diagnostic aid, an office procedure called the Bernstein test, involves anesthetizing the back of the throat, inserting a fine tube, and dripping an acid solution into the esophagus. If reflux is the problem, the acid will produce the typical symptoms. The test is also valuable reassurance for many people that this problem is not more serious.

For many of those with reflux not otherwise helped, a prescription drug, bethanechol, may be valuable. No new agent, bethanechol has been used to overcome postoperative urinary retention because of its ability to contract urinary muscles strongly enough to empty the bladder.

At the U.S. Naval Hospital, Philadelphia, Drs. Donald O. Castell, Raymond L. Farrell, and Gerald T. Roling have shown that the drug can increase LES pressure. And they have reported that 90 percent of patients with previously unyielding heartburn have improved when treated with the drug.

14. When "Nervous" Head Pains, Face Pains, and Headaches Aren't

Headache, it has been said, "is often a complaint of the body against a condition of the mind." And it may be. So, too, many similarly categorized head and face pains. But not invariably; not nearly as often, in fact, as supposed.

Very recently, when a man with chronic head pain appeared in the office of a New York City dentist, he had previously sought help unsuccessfully, he explained, from an internist, a neurologist, a nose and throat specialist, and an orthopedic surgeon.

"How," the dentist wondered, "did you miss seeing a psychiatrist?"

"I'm a psychiatrist myself," the patient announced, "and this is no psychosomatic pain."

It wasn't. Quickly, the dentist could establish and effectively treat what it was: TMJ (temporomandibular joint) dysfunction, a lower-jaw problem.

The same problem is responsible for many misdiagnosed, chronic, unyielding neck and facial pains, seeming earaches, apparent sinus pains, tension headaches, and more.

TMJ dysfunction, which has earned the nickname of "The Great Impostor" because of its ability to produce a wide variety of symptoms and mimic many different diseases, is estimated to affect 20 percent of the population—and is overlooked completely in most.

Its victims, according to Dr. Douglas H. Morgan of White Memorial Medical Center, Los Angeles, "are the persons who go from doctor to doctor with a multitude of seemingly unrelated symptoms. In some, there may be functional problems—an inability to open or close the mouth. In others, there may be only pain that resembles migraine, sinus problems, atypical facial pain mimicking a tic douloureux or a temporal arteritis, or neck and shoulder pain. In others, there may be no pain, only dizziness, tinnitus [ear ringing], or subjective hearing loss."

Reports Dr. Nathan A. Shore, lecturer at the New York University College of Dentistry, who has treated more than 2,800 TMJ patients: "Many have been told they are psychosomatically ill and must learn to live with their 'imaginary' pains. The fact is that it's the pain that makes them neurotic, not neurosis that causes the pain."

Among Shore's patients have been some who have had cranial nerves severed "therapeutically" and some who have had full-mouth extractions of sound sets of teeth in desperate searches for relief.

Just a few years ago, a survey published in the *Journal of the American Dental Association* revealed that "many physicians and dentists still are either uninformed about the syndrome or they are following outdated concepts of diagnosis and treatment for TMJ problems."

How TMJ problems start

The temporomandibular joint, in front of the ear where the lower jaw, or mandible, hinges to the skull, is in almost constant use. We swallow 1,500 to 2,000 times a day, eat three or more meals daily, and talk and form expressions with face and jaw.

Any of a number of causes can lead to trouble in and around the joint.

The jaw can get out of adjustment from a blow to the head

or jaw, or from opening the jaw too wide or too long when biting or yawning.

It can also get out of adjustment in a significant percentage of victims of rear-end auto collisions, Dr. Victor H. Frankel of Case Western Reserve University, Cleveland, has found. In such an accident, the victim's body is accelerated forward, the head is snapped backward, and often the mouth snaps open and shut with great force.

A poor bite can cause trouble. It may develop, for example, when a tooth is lost and that moves the lower jaw out of position, misaligning the joint.

A common cause is clenching or gnashing of the teeth. Dr. Daniel M. Kaskin of the University of Illinois Medical Center, Chicago, reports that such oral habits produce muscle spasm, wear away cusps on the grinding surfaces of teeth, and can force teeth out of alignment. Studies at the Center indicate that some patients with TMJ problems habitually respond to stress by clenching their teeth while other people are more likely to react with increased heartbeat and other signs.

Even such oral habits as nail-biting, excessive gum chewing, or biting of the lip or inner cheek may cause trouble by putting extra stress on the jaw-moving muscles.

Clues amidst the confusion

TMJ dysfunction can, with good reason, be a confusing problem.

Once the joint is affected, the equilibrium of muscles and ligaments that control the joint movement is upset. The muscles then go into spasm, or involuntary contraction, a pain-producing state.

But the pain may radiate a considerable distance, shooting out from little "trigger" areas, small regions of great sensitivity within the muscles.

Trigger areas in the TMJ muscle system can lead to pain, either dull or stabbing, not just around the jaw and teeth but virtually anywhere in the head and in the neck and shoulders.

Yet diagnosis need not be difficult provided the possibility of TMJ dysfunction is considered.

Some patients themselves may have reason to suspect it when they find that their jaw or other pain can be eased by opening the mouth but becomes worse on chewing, speaking, or brushing the teeth; or when they note, upon awakening in the morning, that their jaws are clenched; or when they catch themselves grinding their teeth in moments of concentration.

To help diagnose the TMJ problem, Dr. Shore, who is the author of the standard medical/dental textbook on the subject, *Temporomandibular Joint Dysfunction and Occlusal Equilibration,* has developed simple tests that can be carried out by any physician or dentist in a minute or less.

One involves listening, by ear or with the aid of a stethoscope, for any clicking, or "crepitus," noises (sounds similar to those produced by walking on gravel) when the jaw is moved. Another is simply to note, when the mouth is opened, whether the jaw waves from side to side. And a third involves just feeling, or palpating, the joint on each side with the fingers—and feeling the muscles as well—to detect any spasm.

TMJ treatment measures

Once the joint dysfunction is detected, its treatment may be relatively simple.

A temporary plastic appliance called the Shore Mandibular Autorepositioner, after Dr. Shore, who developed it, has been used successfully on many hundreds of patients. It's a removable biteplate that is fitted to the upper teeth. By keeping the upper teeth separated from the lower, it helps the lower jaw move into proper position and overcomes spasm so the joint gradually begins to function properly.

Except for eating and brushing the teeth, the appliance is worn constantly for about four months. When it is removed, finally, any biting surfaces of teeth that may be contributing to malocclusion are polished.

In some patients, restoration of balance in the use of jaw muscles may be needed. These are people who tend to use only one side of the mouth when chewing. In addition to making a conscious effort to chew on the other side as well, they may be given simple exercises to perform. In one, the tip of the tongue is placed far back on the roof of the mouth and the mouth is then opened wide; this may help to balance the jaw muscles and control crackling. In another, the jaw is moved a given number of times away from the weak side in order to exercise and strengthen the weaker muscles.

For relief of spasm, patients may be advised to apply moist heat for ten minutes at a time, three times a day, to both sides of the face and to eat a soft diet for a time. In some cases, mild analgesics, or pain relievers, along with muscle relaxants may be used temporarily.

The results in previously intractable cases can be striking.

For example, a 38-year-old woman developed a dull, aching pain in the right cheek area which would increase in intensity until the temple throbbed. She likened it to an intermittent headache. Though the pain was slightly less severe at night, she needed frequent medication even then. The highest pain intensity occurred during late afternoon and evening, and often she was unable to control the pain with medication. Sudden weather changes had an adverse effect. Sometimes she could get temporary relief by putting pressure on the cheekbone area or by clenching the inside of her mouth between her teeth and holding that position for several minutes.

Her family physician diagnosed sinus difficulty, but treatment for that didn't help. She had had a wisdom tooth extracted several months before the onset of the pain. During a routine dental examination, an unhealed cleft near the second molar on the upper right side with a portion of bone and tooth root exposed was discovered. The cleft was treated but the pain persisted.

A series of multiple B vitamin injections was tried to no avail. The possibility of tic douloureux, a painful facial nerve disorder, was considered and eliminated. An arthritic condition was considered and eliminated. Cortisone injections failed to relieve the pain.

After a neurological examination disclosed nothing and skull X-rays revealed no abnormalities, the patient was admitted to a hospital for specialized tests. Over a two-week period, she had more X-rays, blood tests, an electroencephalogram, and a lumbar puncture. The results were negative. The pain continued.

Finally, TMJ dysfunction was considered. It was clearly present. It was revealed not only by the simple tests already noted but also showed up clearly on X-rays of the joint. Within six weeks after treatment for the TMJ problem was begun, all pain symptoms disappeared. In five years of follow-up, they have not returned.

One study at the TMJ clinics of the French and Polyclinic Medical School and the New York Eye and Ear Infirmary in New York City included 112 patients with chronic headaches, many diagnosed as migraine. All had been referred from a headache clinic after failure to end the headaches. Some of the patients had other symptoms as well as headaches. All proved to be TMJ victims.

With treatment for the TMJ problem, the headaches improved in all but nine, with sixty-five becoming entirely free of them. Of sixteen who also suffered from vertigo, twelve were helped. Of twenty with ear pain, nineteen benefited, and of thirty-eight with ear noises, all but seven were helped.

In a study at the University of North Carolina Dental School, Chapel Hill, by Dr. Ernest W. Small, forty-nine of fifty patients with deep pain in the side of the face benefited from TMJ treatment.

At the University of Pennsylvania in Philadelphia, Dr. Arnold Gessel has reported on using biofeedback to treat one hundred patients with tension headaches caused by

TMJ dysfunction resulting from jaw clenching. With electrodes attached to their jaw muscles and connected to electronic equipment, patients are able to hear the amplified sounds of muscles contracting and relaxing, the tone getting louder with jaw clenching and softer with relaxation. With practice, they often learn how to keep the muscles relaxed using the equipment as a guide and then subsequently can do so without it. A success rate of 80 percent has been reported.

At the University of Illinois TMJ and Facial Pain Research Center, Dr. Richard J. Dohrmann has used biofeedback for patients with severe facial pain, muscle spasm, jaw clicking, and limited jaw motion. After learning how to relax jaw muscles in thirty-minute, twice-weekly sessions for six weeks, 75 percent of patients have been freed of trouble and have been able to avoid further episodes.

TMJ dysfunction is no newly discovered problem. It has been known and described in the medical and dental literature for forty years. But only very recently has its high incidence—and neglect—become apparent.

Certainly, investigators agree, not all pain or other disturbance that *may* be traceable to TMJ dysfunction necessarily *is*. There can be other causes. But clearly TMJ has to be considered, checked into, and, if found, treated.

In recent years, hospitals and dental schools have begun to set up special clinics for TMJ dysfunction. In many, a team approach is used, with a dentist, ear-nose-and-throat specialist, neurologist, and one or more other specialists working together in the diagnosis and treatment of patients.

The importance of the TMJ condition is finally beginning to be recognized by a broader segment of doctors and dentists. "There is gradually developing a group," says Dr. Morgan of White Memorial, "interested and knowledgeable in this area. More TMJ clinics will be developed in dental schools and hospitals. . . . The future holds more hope for the large numbers afflicted with this severe and perplexing problem."

Other Headaches—Psychogenic and Nonpsychogenic

According to authoritative estimates, some forty million Americans suffer from recurring headaches. The lives of many with the more severe chronic headaches revolve around surviving the pain episodes.

There are, of course, headaches that are known as "secondary": they are symptoms of an underlying organic problem such as head injury, brain tumor, sinus disease, glaucoma, fever, or high blood pressure. And certainly such organic conditions have to be considered in any case of chronic headache.

But by far the most common headaches are the "primary"; those, including migraine and tension headaches, that are not associated with any major illness.

And you've undoubtedly heard it said that the vast majority of such primary headaches are caused by emotional stress.

It has been said, for example, that the most common prelude to migraine is repressed rage and that migraine attacks are "inextricably bound with psychiatric symptoms of life situations or a relatively short-term emotional crisis."

And tension headaches are very commonly held to be the result of just that—psychic tension—although, in fact, the word "tension" as applied to such headaches really refers to muscle tension and many knowledgeable physicians prefer to use the term "muscle contraction" headaches.

Can the common primary headaches be produced by emotional upsets? Undoubtedly. But they don't have to be, and they often may not be.

Although many people, some physicians included, are quick to consider emotional problems to be the cause of headaches, especially when prescribed medications don't work, there are chronic headache victims who suffer little if any significant emotional upset except that which may result from having their frequent headaches.

And among serious headache investigators, the realization has grown that even in those people in whom emotional factors seem to play a basic role in triggering headaches, the real role of emotions sometimes may be no greater, no more of a key factor, than other influences.

Migraine and estrogen

Can oral contraceptives and other preparations containing the hormone estrogen play a role in migraine headaches in some women? So it seems from a study of three hundred patients with migraine carried out by Dr. Lee Kudrow of the California Medical Clinic for Headache in Encino.

According to Dr. Kudrow's report in the medical journal *Headache,* the estrogen-containing Pill and other estrogen-containing medications often increased headache frequency. Moreover, they led to migrainelike headaches in some nonmigrainous women. And with elimination or reduction in dosage of the estrogen-containing preparations, a significant reduction in headache attack frequency occurred.

Migraine and diet

In their efforts to avoid repeated attacks, many migraine sufferers have resorted to various diets, some of them bizarre.

Yet, despite many misconceptions about diet and migraine, reports Dr. Donald J. Dalessio of the Scripps Clinic and Research Foundation, La Jolla, California, some dietary measures may be helpful in many cases.

Certain foods can, in the migraine-prone, have an effect on blood vessels that may lead to attacks. They include red wines and champagne, aged or strong cheese (particularly Cheddar), pickled herring, chicken livers, pods of broad beans, and canned figs. Avoidance of them may be useful.

In some cases, cured meats, including frankfurters,

bacon, ham, and salami, may have adverse effects and a trial of avoiding them may be worthwhile.

Monosodium glutamate in excessive amounts may trigger migraine and should be avoided.

And it is also important for migraine sufferers to avoid hypoglycemia, or low blood sugar. For this reason, Dr. Dalessio recommends, they should eat three well-balanced meals a day, avoiding excessive amounts of sugar and starches at any one meal.

Recently, too, another investigator has found that salted snack foods, such as pretzels, potato chips, and nuts, particularly if taken on an empty stomach, may trigger a migraine episode within six to twelve hours. Dr. John B. Brainard of St. Paul, Minnesota, had a dozen patients, all with long histories of migraine, record the incidence of attacks both before and after avoiding salted snack foods before meals. In ten of the twelve, the salt restriction led to significant reductions in the number of headaches.

The platelet abnormality in migraine

Unexpectedly, a few years ago, physicians prescribing a drug, propranolol, for patients with heart problems found that some who also happened to be migraine sufferers soon reported a marked decrease in headache episodes.

There followed studies to check on this. In one, two University of Miami neurologists, Drs. R. B. Weber and O. M. Reinmuth, chose a group of patients with unyielding migraine, failures on other treatment. For three months, each patient received propranolol in 20 milligram doses four times a day; for another three months, for comparison, the patients got identical-looking but inert medication.

Propranolol turned out to be clearly valuable in many. The response of one-third of the group was rated excellent, with complete disappearance of migraine episodes after one week of treatment. Another 50 percent had a good response, with 50 percent or greater reduction in severity or frequency of attacks.

Why? What does propranolol do to combat migraine?

The blood contains tiny ovoid bodies called platelets which under specific circumstances serve a valuable purpose. When there is a break in a blood vessel wall leading to bleeding, the platelets, which have been circulating in the blood, clump together at the break site and initiate clot formation to plug the break and stop the bleeding.

Recent studies in patients with coronary heart disease suggest that part of their problem, perhaps an important part, is altered or accelerated platelet aggregation, a tendency for platelets to clump together when that is not called for. And some studies have shown that propranolol restores platelet aggregation toward normal.

Within just the last several years, a series of studies has indicated that there are abnormalities of platelet aggregation in patients with migraine. Propranolol's effectiveness in reducing or preventing migraine attacks could well be due to its activity in restoring platelet aggregation toward normal.

Other drugs as well have been found to be effective as platelet antagonists. They include dipyridamole, sulfinpyrazone, and fenoprofen calcium. Many of these agents are currently being evaluated in coronary heart disease. And preliminary studies at the Scripps Clinic and Research Foundation suggest that sulfinpyrazone and fenoprofen may be particularly effective in reducing the frequency and intensity of migraine attacks.

Tension headache

Tension headache is the most common type of headache. It is often described as a squeezing pain around the back of the head, forehead, scalp, and neck. The pain is usually constant but sometimes may become jabbing.

As indicated earlier, tension headache is more accurately

called muscle contraction headache. It arises from spasm, or contraction, of neck, face, and scalp muscles.

What provokes the spasm? Certainly, emotional factors can. Fear, frustration, worry, anxiety often may be involved. It has been said of many sufferers that they "symbolically carry a great weight on their shoulders." Upon feeling upset, they set scalp, neck, and face muscles and develop headache.

But nonemotional influences also are capable of leading to spasm.

Pain almost anywhere in the body—in the teeth, in the neck, or at a more distant site—can lead to contraction of headache-producing muscles.

Muscle contraction headache often accompanies arthritis of the neck area of the spine. It can be triggered by a neck injury, or by poor posture with the head or neck maintained in an awkward position for a prolonged period.

Recurrent muscle contraction headaches deserve a careful medical check rather than a glib assumption that they are simply a matter of emotions. Even when obvious emotional upset is present, the headaches can be the result not of the upset alone but of a physical problem that makes it easier for the upset to trigger spasm and pain.

Treatment for the headaches may include one or more of a number of drugs. In some cases, simple analgesics such as aspirin and acetaminophen are of use. Tranquilizers may be prescribed because, beyond their tranquilizing activity, such drugs as Valium, Librium, and Miltown, for example, also have muscle-relaxing properties.

Many patients are helped by heat and massage, by special collars to help maintain good posture, by neck muscle exercises, by sleeping on a neck-supporting pillow.

Weekend and holiday headaches

Weekend and holiday headaches are often blamed on emotional factors—on inability to relax, on the need to keep busy. The blame may be valid in many cases but not necessarily so in many others.

Some recent studies suggest, for example, that some people are accustomed to consuming large amounts of caffeine-containing beverages beginning early in the morning on weekdays. They are accustomed to the vasoconstrictive, or blood vessel narrowing, effect of caffeine. When they sleep later on holidays and weekends, the early-morning caffeine deprivation may lead to a widening of blood vessels, which can cause headache.

Alternatively, without regard to caffeine, holiday and weekend headaches may stem from increased REM sleep at these times because of longer sleeping periods. Headaches that begin during sleep have been found to do so during REM.

Cured-meat headaches

Nitrites are chemicals often used as preservatives in cured meats. They also act as color fixers, helping to keep the meats looking red and fresh.

Sensitivity to nitrites in some people may be responsible for otherwise mysterious headaches that might be attributed too readily to emotional disturbances.

In one case that came under special study, a 58-year-old man had been experiencing for seven years moderately severe, nonthrobbing headaches that usually lasted several hours and were sometimes accompanied by facial flushing. Finally, it became apparent that the attacks developed within half an hour after he ate such cured-meat products as frankfurters, bacon, salami, and ham.

Since no other foods or beverages produced the headaches and he was not otherwise prone to headaches, tests to determine whether the nitrites in the cured-meat products might be the culprits were carried out by Drs. William R. Handerson and Neil H. Raskin of the University of California, San Francisco, Department of Neurology.

For the tests, the patient drank odorless, tasteless solutions that sometimes contained 10 milligrams of sodium nitrite and at other times contained the same amount of sodium bicarbonate. Headaches were provoked eight out of the thirteen times he drank the sodium nitrite.

Bedcover ("turtle") headaches

Bedcovers may seem an unlikely cause of puzzling headaches, or, more accurately, sleeping with bedcovers pulled up over the head.

But, writing in the *Journal of the American Medical Association* not long ago, Dr. Gordon J. Gilbert of St. Petersburg, Florida, reported on a series of patients suffering from such headaches. His pet name for them: turtle headaches.

They may wake the victim during the night or may be present on awakening in the morning. They may be generalized, with pain all over the head, but usually are most painful in front of the head.

They are accounted for, Dr. Gilbert suggests, by oxygen shortage, resulting from pulling the covers well up over the head. In his experience, once the cover-up habit is eliminated, so, immediately, are the headaches.

Between-meals headaches

Headaches are among the symptoms that may be caused by hypoglycemia, or abnormally low blood sugar. But, without being hypoglycemic, some people develop headaches if they go for long periods, most often longer than five hours, between meals, even though their blood sugar may not get down to abnormally low levels. The solution, of course, is more and smaller meals.

Toxic headaches

Headaches, usually moderate and generalized, can be produced by many chemical compounds.

Among the most common culprits are such organic solvents as turpentine, carbon tetrachloride, benzine in gasoline, and benzene.

Carbon monoxide can cause headaches and not infrequently is responsible for them in automobile mechanics or others working in atmospheres where carbon monoxide may rise to excessive levels.

Drug headaches

Many drugs are capable of causing headaches as side effects in some people who happen to be sensitive.

Among them are even some tranquilizing agents such as Equanil, Miltown, and Valium.

Antihistamine drugs such as Benadryl, Chlor-Trimeton, and Periactin can be responsible for headaches. So, too, a variety of agents used for high blood pressure, including Aldactazide, Aldomet, Hydrodiuril, Reserpine, and Ser-Ap-Es, and also even some used to relieve pain, such as Demerol and Indocin, the latter often employed for arthritic pain.

In fact, so many drugs can, in the occasional patient, produce headache that if you begin to suffer from headaches not long after your physician has prescribed a drug for any purpose, it could be well to check with him on the possibility that it is the source of headache.

15. *Senile Dementia: Healthy New Holes in a Wastebasket Diagnosis*

The situation has been all too familiar. The patient is elderly—or sometimes only middle-aged. His behavior has become bizarre. He is increasingly forgetful and slovenly. He may be irritable and suspicious as well. His family has been brought to the point of despair.

More often than not, when medical help has been sought, the diagnosis has been senile dementia if the patient is old, presenile dementia if middle-aged, attributable to hardening of the brain arteries, with nothing to be done except perhaps institutionalization.

The scenario was strikingly different, however, when a 66-year-old man was brought to Mount Sinai Hospital in New York. Two years before, he had first experienced an episode of confusion, disorientation, and severe headache lasting several hours. Subsequently, he had gradually deteriorated, his personality changing markedly toward suspiciousness. Two months before hospital admission, he fell without losing consciousness and then deteriorated very rapidly.

On admission, he was confused, disoriented, had memory deficits, anxiety, depression, marked paranoid suspiciousness, and was incontinent of urine and feces.

Forty-eight hours later, after surgery to correct hydrocephalus ("water on the brain"), he was alert, cheerful, oriented, free of paranoid thinking and incontinence.

The discovery that hydrocephalus can be responsible for at least some cases of senile dementia is one of the more dramatic examples of new developments in an area that has badly needed them.

Too often, senile dementia has been a wastebasket diagnosis—in reality, no diagnosis at all but an easy disposal category. There has been a pronounced tendency to link behavioral changes in older people with just one thing: hardening of brain arteries. And there has been a pervasive pessimism and often a do-nothingism, the argument being that hardening of brain arteries cannot be reversed and hence nothing could be done for the behavioral changes that could only get worse.

Yet senility is not invariably linked with artery hardening. Many manifestations of mental "deterioration" have nothing to do with artery hardening or even other brain disease. They can be precipitated by physical problems, deprivations, and insults far removed from the brain, and these are often controllable and in some cases even curable.

Moreover, even when there is hardening of brain arteries, the situation may be far from hopeless. Other factors may be contributing to the behavioral problems. Those factors include infections, injuries, drug intoxication, nutritional deficiencies, heart conditions—virtually all of those discussed elsewhere in this book.

"Perhaps the greatest of all [pitfalls]," observes one expert in geriatric medicine, Dr. William Reichel of Franklin Square Hospital, Baltimore, "is stereotyping the elderly patient as the victim of 'aging' or arteriosclerosis, obviously irreversible processes. This excuses us from compiling and analyzing the problems about which the patient complains and from considering the differential diagnoses. Somewhere along the line, treatable problems may be passed over."

The occult hydrocephalus phenomenon

That hydrocephalus, or water on the brain, occurs in some children has long been known. When it does, it is obvious. It is not obvious in the same way in an adult.

Within the brain are four fluid-containing reservoirs, the ventricles. In effect, the reservoirs float the brain on fluid, an excellent shock-absorber mechanism. The brain, of course, is part of the central nervous system, which includes the spinal cord. The cord too is surrounded by shock-cushioning fluid.

When the normal flow of cerebrospinal fluid is impaired by a congenital malformation, fluid accumulates in the brain and enlarges the ventricles. This is hydrocephalus, which in a child causes enlargement of the cranium.

In a hydrocephalic child, fluid is trapped in the ventricles, which become distended. The distention makes the child's still-soft skull bones spread and the head balloons grotesquely. Most cases begin soon after birth or during infancy and if unchecked may lead to mental and physical deterioration as well as massive head enlargement.

Surgery for hydrocephalus in a child diverts fluid around an obstruction and into the blood circulation. A fine tube is inserted through a small scalp incision and burr hole in the skull into a ventricle and is threaded under the scalp and under the skin of the neck to the jugular vein, then down through the vein to the heart. This is a ventriculoatrial shunt, or bypass, and, by re-establishing fluid flow, it can work wonders for a child.

But hydrocephalus in an elderly patient does not produce head enlargement and it need not even be marked by increased pressure. The first report from a Harvard Medical School team that pioneered investigation and treatment of adult hydrocephalus was on three elderly patients without head enlargement and without increase of pressure within the brain.

One was a 63-year-old woman whose illness started with an episode of weakness, giddiness, and pallor from which she recovered the following day. Thereafter, however, she tired easily, became forgetful, less able to concentrate and organize her daily affairs, lost urinary control, and was uncertain of gait.

Six months after onset of her illness, she entered Massachusetts General Hospital, a Harvard teaching institution in Boston. Among many studies performed, there was one for cerebrospinal fluid pressure and another involving skull X-rays. Both were normal. But a special X-ray of the brain after injection of air—a pneumoencephalogram—revealed massive enlargement of the ventricle system. Very soon after a shunt operation, performed much as for a child with hydrocephalus, she began to improve and continued to improve. Three years later, at age 66, her intellectual performance in standard tests was graded "superior," her memory "very superior."

There were equally striking results in the other two patients, one of whom was a 62-year-old pediatrician with a six-month history of increasing slowness of thought and action, forgetfulness, unsteadiness of gait, and incontinence. He was able to return to practice after surgery.

Results reported from many other medical centers recently have been excellent. Today, too, newer diagnostic techniques, including CAT (computerized axial tomography), facilitate the detection of occult hydrocephalus.

What causes it? It may occur following head injury, hemorrhage, meningitis, or brain tumor. But it may also occur for unknown reasons in patients who have had none of these.

Shunting is not a minor procedure and, as with any surgery, entails some risk of infection and other possible complications. But when suitably used, it can avoid vegetation for many patients for whom until very recently the outlook was hopeless.

Thinning the blood

A seemingly senile 81-year-old woman lay in a Pittsburgh hospital bed staring blankly about her, unable to sign her name, fervently clutching a stuffed dog. Several weeks later, she wrote a note of gratitude for what had happened and put away the dog.

What had happened, the relief of her seeming senility symptoms, was achieved by use of a new form of treatment for senile and presenile dementia developed by Dr. Arthur C. Walsh, a psychiatrist who is clinical assistant professor at the University of Pittsburgh and psychiatric consultant at the Veterans Administration Hospital and the Western Psychiatric Institute and Clinic in Pittsburgh.

The treatment combines doses of a drug, an anticoagulant, with psychotherapy. At a recent annual American Psychiatric Association meeting in Toronto, Walsh presented the findings of a two-year study of forty-nine patients with senile or presenile dementia, thirty-four of whom had improved significantly on the combination treatment.

Nearly all patients in the series, Walsh reported, had failed to respond to previous treatment elsewhere and regarded the new treatment program as a last resort. Many were deteriorated to the point of being unable to carry on a semblance of normal conversation. After four months of anticoagulant-psychotherapy treatment, those who benefited were able to function almost or entirely on their own.

The reasoning behind the treatment is that a major cause of senility may be blood sludging, or aggregation of red blood cells. Some years ago, Dr. M. H. Knisely of the Medical University of South Carolina noted that narrowing of blood vessels in aging can cause red cells to adhere and form aggregations that impair blood flow.

Knisely had also pointed out that diabetes and alcoholism, among other conditions, can cause blood sludging. And in early work, Walsh studied fifteen alcohol-brain-damaged patients, of whom twelve responded to anticoagulant treatment after other treatment methods had failed. The anticoagulant acted against the sludging.

Blood sludging, Walsh considered, could represent a pre-clot formation phenomenon, and while it could arise from blood vessel constriction causing a slowdown in blood flow, a contributory factor could be emotional stress causing extra adrenaline release that increased the clotting tendency. Therefore, psychotherapy might be in order.

In psychotherapy, Walsh encourages a patient to "review his life." This, he believes, serves a purpose even beyond reducing emotional stress. It "stimulates brain cells that are still alive but not functioning." In fact, Walsh sees life-reviewing as "the mental exercise equivalent to physiotherapy used to strengthen arms and legs after the motor areas of the brain are damaged by a stroke."

In early trials, Walsh used Dicumarol as the anticoagulant. Later he changed to Coumadin because it is easier to control and because most doctors are familiar with its use.

If improvement occurs, Walsh recommends continued anticoagulant use indefinitely. In the studies, half of the patients who had improved began to regress when taken off anticoagulant. Relatives are instructed in how to handle anticoagulant much as patients and relatives learn to handle insulin for diabetes.

Anticoagulant treatment for senility must still be considered experimental. Before it is generally accepted, many physicians will have to test it. Such testing has begun. At Maimonides Hospital and Home for the Aged, Montreal, investigators studied two comparable groups of patients with advanced senile dementia, half of whom received anticoagulant treatment while the others, for comparison, received inert medication (placebo). In the placebo group, after a year, the mean memory quotient declined by two-thirds; in those receiving anticoagulant, the decline was about 10 percent. Tests for other characteristics revealed markedly greater deterioration in the placebo group. The Canadian investigators, believing the treatment would have been more effective if earlier cases had been chosen, have begun a study with a larger group of patients.

Dilating blood vessels

Efforts to improve the lot of the senile have included use of drugs to dilate blood vessels.

One of these drugs is a tablet called Hydergine. Animal studies have indicated that it has an ability to dilate brain blood vessels. There are also indications that it may reduce blood vessel resistance to blood flow and possibly also improve utilization of oxygen.

In one study, patients aged 59 to 95 received either 0.5 milligram of Hydergine or a placebo, administered under the tongue, six times a day for twelve weeks. The treated patients improved markedly by the end of the first month and continued to show improvement through the third month, with no undesirable side effects. They experienced less dizziness, ate better, had improved coordination, and tended to be less agitated and to tremble less, in marked contrast to those receiving placebo.

A double-blind study was carried out in a Massachusetts home for the aged. In such a study, some patients receive the medication being tested while others get a placebo, and neither patients nor physicians know who is receiving what until the trial is over. The objective is to eliminate any effects of hopefulness and enthusiasm engendered by taking part in a trial and also by physicians' attitudes and enthusiasms.

The Massachusetts study included forty elderly patients with cerebrovascular disorders. Among them were patients with mental deterioration diagnosed as due to cerebral arteriosclerosis or senile cerebral degeneration. In the twelve-week study, Hydergine relieved a number of manifestations of cerebrovascular insufficiency, including inability to perform basic self-care tasks, some physical complaints, some aspects of mood and attitude, and intellectual deterioration. Patients receiving the real medication showed improvement in appetite, headache complaints, emotional instability, anxiety and fears, ability to follow instructions, confusion, and memory defect.

Clearly, Hydergine is far from a specific treatment for senility, but it may be helpful for at least some patients.

Meanwhile, in England, at Powick Hospital, Worcestershire, Dr. Peter Hall has been carrying out a study with another drug, cyclandelate, that dilates blood vessels and may help to improve blood flow to the brain. A first report covers twenty-one patients, aged to 88, who sometimes received the drug and at other times a look-alike but inert preparation.

During active drug treatment, improvement occurred in mental state, mood, orientation, memory, and abstraction. "Cyclandelate and perhaps other drugs—together with supportive and rehabilitative measures—offer some hope," reports Hall, "of improving the ability of these patients to cope with their everyday life in terms of memory, comprehension, and manual dexterity."

Artery surgery

Out of the surgical treatment of little strokes in order to prevent big strokes recently has come new hope for some patients with senility.

Before a paralyzing or deadly stroke, many people have momentary episodes of stumbling, numbness or paralysis of a hand, vision blurring, or speech or memory loss, indicative of reduced blood flow to the brain.

Until relatively recently, it was believed that most obstructions reducing flow and leading to stroke occurred in arteries buried within the brain and unreachable by surgery. Recent studies, however, indicate that as many as 74 percent of patients have at least one lesion in a surgically accessible site. Often the site is a carotid artery at the side of the neck, a major avenue of blood circulation to the brain.

Carotid endarterectomy, a procedure in which a carotid artery is opened and the obstruction surgically scraped out, has been found valuable, relieving symptoms in most cases and markedly reducing the incidence of subsequent massive strokes, and endarterectomy is now often used.

Very recently, the possibility has been opened up that carotid endarterectomy may do more than prevent strokes, that it may improve mental abilities, according to Dr. C.

Doyle Haynes of Emory University School of Medicine, Atlanta.

In the course of doing endarterectomies, Haynes had gotten an impression from the postoperative course of many patients that their mental status improved. More than an impression was needed, however.

Working with psychologists from Auburn University, Dr. Haynes managed to compare the preoperative and postoperative mental conditions of seventeen endarterectomy patients and to compare, further, any changes in them with what happened in eight surgical patients who had no evidence of artery-hardening disease. Patients in both groups took psychological tests within twenty-four hours before their operations and the tests were repeated between four and eight weeks later.

As expected, both groups of patients were anxious prior to going into the operating room and both were less scared six weeks later. But, beyond that, the endarterectomy patients had less "trait" anxiety—meaning chronic predisposition to feeling anxious—after surgery than before while the others remained almost exactly the same.

Other interesting changes measured by psychological tests turned up only in the endarterectomy group. These patients had lower postoperative scores for confusion, disorientation, and suspicion. They also had higher average scores in both verbal and perceptual IQ tests after surgery, many of them adding up to as much as 22.5 points on verbal tests and 35.1 on perceptual tests.

Almost at the same time as Dr. Haynes was reporting his work, another study was reported by Dr. Gary G. Ferguson, assistant professor of neurosurgery, University Hospital, London, Ontario.

Ferguson had worked with a series of ten patients with dementia. The average period of dementia was six months although two patients had shown symptoms for more than two years. The average age of the patients, all of whom were men, was 60 years. All had experienced minor strokes. It turned out that all had more than one artery blockage or severe narrowing.

Ferguson chose to try to get more blood to the brain by connecting two ordinarily separated arteries, the superficial temporal artery and the cortical arterial branch of the middle cerebral artery, and thus feeding brain areas deprived of adequate blood supply.

All the patients had been severely disabled before the operation. None had been able to work; two had been institutionalized. After surgery, the two patients who had shown signs of dementia for more than two years returned to work and three others were able to work on a limited basis; four others showed some improvement as judged by their families; and one was unimproved.

Seeming senility from other causes

"Sophie E, 73, is confused, disoriented, frightened. Although she was alert and independent just days before, her physician settles on a diagnosis of chronic irreversible brain syndrome, a progressive disease that takes years to develop. The viral infection that caused Sophie's bout of confusion is never discovered, and she is admitted to a nursing home.

"Max H, 86, also is confused and disoriented. His physician tells Max's family that such behavior is to be expected in a man of his advanced years. He never realizes that Max has suffered a heart attack—without the chest pains, shortness of breath and other classic symptoms.

"Jean S, 75, complains of malaise and appears confused when she appears for a regular physical. Her physician sends her home with a prescription for a tranquilizer and assurance that a woman of her age shouldn't expect 'to feel like a spring chicken.' But Jean's symptoms are due, not to age, but to appendicitis, again without such classic symptoms as abdominal tenderness, fever and a high white blood count."

These three cases were published recently in the medical publication *The New Physician*. Rare phenomena? It is to be hoped that these misdiagnoses are, or soon will become, rare, but such instances of mental change in older people brought on by these and other physical diseases are not rare.

"The tragedy of health care for the aged," *The New Physician* observed, "is that doctors in this country often don't know what signs and symptoms to look for in their elderly patients. The reason they don't know is simple: no one ever told them. But medicine's traditional indifference to geriatric care is approaching a crisis point. The 'graying' of America demands that tomorrow's doctors learn how to care for elderly patients."

Physicians who have made care of the elderly a special concern are trying now to educate not only tomorrow's doctors but today's as well. And a major point they try to make in their educational efforts is that physical disease in the elderly often presents as mental disorder.

Emphasizes Dr. William Reichel: "... because of the compromises in brain function that accompany aging, elderly patients tend to show confusion and disorientation as a first sign of infection, pneumonia, cardiac failure, coronary occlusion, electrolyte imbalance, anemia, or dehydration. The brain changes may have no behavioral expression at all in the absence of major stress. The presumption of senility or 'chronic brain syndrome' is unwarranted in the context of sudden behavioral change; rather, we may be dealing with the behavioral concomitants of a reversible medical illness or drug toxicity."

In a recent series of reports to physicians, Dr. Reichel has cited many illustrative cases.

As an example of behavioral changes due to drug toxicity: A 66-year-old woman was hospitalized after several days of increasing confusion, disorientation, weakness, nausea, and depression. She was found to be taking a variety of drugs: for diabetes, infection, high blood pressure, plus a major tranquilizer as well. All drugs were withdrawn. On discharge, she showed no need for any of the drugs. Her confusion and other symptoms had disappeared.

As an example of another cause of behavioral changes: An 80-year-old businessman, still active as president of his own corporation, had to be hospitalized after several days of increasing confusion and excitability. He was unable to give doctors a clear history. Studies showed a low level of oxygen in his arterial blood and a lung scan indicated a high probability of pulmonary embolism (a clot lodged in a lung vessel). After a course of an anticoagulant, heparin, for the clot, blood oxygen levels improved, breathing became normal, and mental confusion cleared.

As an example of still another reversible cause of confusion: A 75-year-old retired executive, active as grandfather, sports enthusiast, and churchman, was brought to a physician after several days of increasing confusion, agitation, and memory loss. When he was examined thoroughly, a lung X-ray revealed pneumonia. After ten days of treatment with penicillin injections, his mental functions returned to normal as his pneumonia cleared.

Almost any factor that reduces the flow of oxygen-rich blood to the brain may be involved in senility. Such factors include congestive heart failure, anemia, high blood pressure, and excessive thyroid function, either independently or in combination.

In congestive heart failure, the heart does not stop; rather, it loses some of its pumping efficiency. It may do so as the result of anemia because, with anemia reducing the amount of oxygen carried in the blood, the heart tries to compensate, pumping harder and more often to circulate more blood. High blood pressure increases the work load of the heart. And excessive thyroid function stimulates the heart abnormally. After years of responding to such demands, the heart loses some of its pumping strength. It pumps less blood. The heart may not completely empty. Pressure then builds up within the heart.

The pressure is transmitted back to the lungs, causing shortness of breath. The kidneys, no longer supplied adequately with blood, no longer produce normal urine output and the volume of water in the blood increases and adds to congestion in the lungs. Pressure may also extend backward from the heart to the vein system so that less blood returns to the heart and fluid accumulates in body tissues, swelling ankles and abdomen. Meanwhile, the brain blood supply also suffers.

Vigorous treatment for congestive heart failure aims at three things: to improve the heart's pumping efficiency; to eliminate excess fluids; and to reduce the overload on the heart, immediately if necessary by bed rest, and where possible by treatment of the condition that led to failure.

To improve pumping efficiency, the drug digitalis is often used. The dosage of digitalis must be tailored carefully to the needs of the individual patient. Inadequate doses do little if any good. Excessive doses may cause varied disturbances, including nausea, vomiting, diarrhea, appetite loss, vision blurring, headache, lethargy, and numbness. With effective digitalis therapy, heart performance may improve enough so that even if the condition that caused the failure cannot be corrected, blood can be pumped efficiently.

To eliminate excess fluid, other measures also may be used. Reduction of salt in the diet helps because salt tends to hold water in the body. Diuretic drugs, which act to rid the body of excess fluids, are often valuable.

Once heart failure is overcome, proper care often can help prevent recurrence. Necessary care will vary from one person to another. It may include continued use of digitalis and a diuretic, and limitation of salt intake. And it may include efforts to reduce the overload on the heart. This may call, for example, for correcting anemia. Often it should include control of high blood pressure, which commonly contributes to failure.

Uncontrolled high blood pressure apparently has another undesirable contribution to make to the problems of the elderly. Evidence of its effects on the intellect has been observed in a Duke University study of 202 men and women in their 60's and 70's over a ten-year period. At the beginning and at intervals thereafter, each man and woman had blood pressure taken and was given a battery of intelligence tests.

The study showed that over the ten years, those who had normal pressures experienced no intellectual decline while those with elevated pressures had drops of almost ten points in test scores.

"The purpose of our study," reported Dr. Carl Eisdorfer, who headed the research, "is to demythologize the aging process, which is full of misconceptions. The more we accept intellectual deterioration as inevitable, the less likely we are to do anything about preventing it."

Hypertension today is a correctable problem.

Presenile dementia is conventionally defined as dementia beginning before the age of 65. It can produce defects of recent memory, disorientation, confusion, apathetic withdrawal from social contact, and defects of calculation and speech.

And in a recent report on such dementia, Dr. Maurice H. Charlton, associate professor of neurology at the University of Rochester School of Medicine and Dentistry, emphasized that it has numerous possible causes and that a significant number of remediable causes can be uncovered by adequate study.

One cause, for example, can be a subdural hematoma, a mass of coagulated blood between the tough casing and the more delicate membranes of the brain. A patient with a subdural hematoma need not have a history of significant head injury and there may be no loss of consciousness. Instead, the symptoms may be confined to personality changes.

Similarly, Dr. Charlton noted, underfunctioning of the thyroid gland or vitamin B_{12} deficiency may appear primarily as dementia without any of the classical signs and symptoms of those disorders.

Various drugs—among them, bromides and barbiturates, and perhaps some of the newer tranquilizing and other psychotropic drugs even in mild doses in susceptible people—may cause dementia which disappears when the drugs are withdrawn.

There are, of course, causes for dementia, senile and presenile, that are difficult or impossible to treat—advanced hardening of arteries within the brain and certain diseases such as Alzheimer's and Pick's, which produce abnormal changes in areas of the brain.

But the conclusion from recent studies seems clear enough: too often, dementia has been regarded as a hopeless condition when quite often it is not.

16. Nutritional-Behavioral Links

- In 1937, Dr. Conrad Elvehjem, then a young University of Wisconsin College of Agriculture instructor, isolated from liver extract a nicotinelike chemical. He called it nicotinic acid and in an early experiment found that it could cure—and prevent—blacktongue in dogs. And blacktongue is a dog version of pellagra.

  Quickly, nicotinic acid, to become known also as niacin and vitamin B_3, proved to be the specific cure and preventive for human pellagra.

  But the discovery had much greater significance. Relatively common in the U.S. South, pellagra involved rough skin and diarrhea. But it also was characterized by dementia.

  Recognition that a nutrient deficiency could trigger a psychiatric disorder and that making up the deficiency could cure it was to give tremendous impetus to modern biological psychiatry, which holds that some, perhaps many, mental disturbances have organic rather than psychological roots.
- For fifty-six days in 1973, six conscientious objectors served as volunteers in a study at the U.S. Army Medical Research and Nutrition Laboratory at Fitzsimmons General Hospital, Denver. They lived on a diet adequate in

every way except one: it was deficient in the vitamin riboflavin.

Even before the end of the experiment, the men began to show major personality changes, becoming depressed and hypochondriacal, and even verging toward hysteria. Clearly, riboflavin had effects on behavior.

In 1976, when an international conference was held at the University of Montreal on the role of another nutrient, magnesium, in health, a University of Pretoria, South Africa, team had a striking report to make.

In the course of their magnesium investigations, they had been impressed by the low blood levels of magnesium in some patients seeking medical help for insomnia, tension, and anxiety.

In a trial with two hundred such patients, they had studied the effects of a daily intake of eight 250-milligram tablets of magnesium chloride. In 99 percent of the patients, sleep was rapidly induced and uninterrupted, and waking tiredness disappeared. At the same time, anxiety and tension also diminished.

We are, right now, in the midst—or perhaps more accurately at the beginning—of a revolution in medical thinking about nutrition and the impact of even marginal deficiencies in many areas of health, including the mental and behavioral.

Much recent research has been indicating not only that mental and behavioral upsets can result from nutritional deficiencies but that often they are the first manifestations of marginal deficiencies—and that marginal deficiencies are not rarities.

The stages of deficiency

Nutritional deficiencies and their manifestations don't develop suddenly and acutely. Five different stages of depletion have been identified.

In the first, not enough of a nutrient is available. That

may be because of inadequate intake in the diet. It may also result from malabsorption problems that interfere with the body's uptake of the nutrient. Or it can occur because of certain drugs that interfere with utilization. In this stage, tissue stores of the nutrient are gradually depleted.

If the first stage continues, a second—biochemical—stage follows. Now tissue stores are reduced sufficiently to retard body biochemical activities for which the nutrient is essential.

In the third stage, the tissue depletion and biochemical slowing reach a point of producing behavioral manifestations. There may be appetite loss, general malaise, sleeping difficulty, irritability. Neurotic scores turn up on personality tests.

Later, in the fourth stage, with deficiency still progressing, there are increased behavioral changes, and now, too, physical disturbances that vary with the particular nutrient. For example, if the deficiency is of the vitamin thiamine, there may be leg swelling and pain on walking, heart enlargement, and slowing of the heartbeat.

Finally, the fifth, or terminal, stage is one in which total nutritional depletion can become so severe that serious physical changes occur and death may follow unless the nutrient is restored.

Dr. Myron Brin of the Roche Research Center, one of the chief investigators of marginal deficiency, considers that it comprises the first three stages of depletion.

Brin reported to a 1977 American Chemical Society symposium on marginal deficiency that such deficiency is one in which a person can be otherwise apparently normal according to many of the physical diagnosis procedures carried out in a physician's office.

"But," he emphasized, "due to tissue depletion there are biochemical changes . . . reflected in behavioral changes [which] may influence the productivity of the individual in society, whether he be a child at school, a young adult at college, or an older person earning a living.

"It should be noted," Brin also took pains to point out,

"that these behavioral changes . . . are usually no different from changes which may occur as a consequence of various forms of emotional and physiological stress, and/or social trauma."

The incidence of marginal deficiencies

In the mid-1960's, nutritional studies carried out in Syracuse and in Onondaga County, New York, among two groups in the population, adolescents and the elderly, found inadequacies of vitamins A, B_1, and C.

Later, these findings were confirmed and extended for the whole United States by a variety of nutritional status surveys by federal government agencies, including the U.S. Department of Agriculture Market Basket Survey of 1965, the Department of Health, Education, and Welfare Ten State Nutrition Survey done between 1970 and 1972, and a more recent HANES (Health and Nutrition Examination Survey) of the Department of Health, Education, and Welfare.

The Ten State Survey, for example, examined, among other intakes, the adequacy of intake of the vitamin riboflavin and discovered that 17 percent of Americans below the poverty level were low in riboflavin. But the deficiency was not limited to the poor. An incidence in the neighborhood of about 8 percent was discovered in better-off Americans.

Recently, a special Clinical Nutrition Research Unit team of physicians was organized at the University of Cape Town, South Africa. A major aim of the Unit is to help physicians diagnose nutritional diseases in complicated cases.

The team decided to look into thiamine deficiency in hospital patients. And when they blood-tested for the vitamin, they found 43 percent of a group of patients with deficiency. In some cases, alcoholism was the presumptive cause. In many cases, there were other causes, including ulcer, gastroenteritis, malabsorption, and fasting because of obesity. The team then looked into the thiamine status of children being treated in the outpatient department for gastroenteritis. Fifteen percent were deficient.

In a 1974 study reported in the *American Journal of Clinical Nutrition,* when the status of 599 expectant American mothers was checked, more than 25 percent were found to be thiamine-depleted.

World Health Organization studies indicate that deficiency of another vitamin, folic acid, occurs in one-third to one-half of all pregnant women throughout the world and studies in the United States have shown that American women are no exceptions.

In a British study of fifty-nine elderly psychiatric cases newly admitted to hospital, forty-eight were found to have subnormal folic acid blood levels. In another, low levels were found in thirty-seven of seventy-five psychiatric patients.

A study conducted at the University of Illinois in 1977 found that older persons who have such symptoms as forgetfulness, apathy, depression, and psychosis often have low blood levels of folic acid.

And recently, because of mounting evidence indicating that many diets are deficient now in ten nutrients—vitamin A, thiamine, riboflavin, niacin, B_6, folic acid, iron, calcium, magnesium, and zinc—the Food and Nutrition Board of the National Research Council has urged that many foods be enriched with these materials.

The behavioral effects of deficiencies of many of these nutrients have been coming under study.

Thiamine (vitamin B_1)

At the University of Minnesota some years ago, Dr. J. Brozek studied the psychological effects of thiamine inadequacy in normal young men. He found large changes in the direction of deterioration on the psychoneurotic scales of the Minnesota Multiphasic Personality Inventory. Later, these changes were reversed with thiamine supplements.

And the personality changes, Brozek noted, appeared before such other symptoms as gastric distress, weight loss, and abnormal tingling and burning sensations that thiamine deficiency may produce.

Other investigators have reported that thiamine-deficiency-associated disturbances may include irritability, memory impairment, depression, difficulty in concentration, and confusion, all of which can come from many other problems but when associated with thiamine deficiency clear up when thiamine is administered.

Alcoholics are particularly prone to thiamine deficiency not only because they may eat less of foods containing the vitamin but also because they have subnormal absorption. But thiamine deficiency can affect almost anyone. The adult daily requirement is in the range of only 1 to 1½ milligrams, but the total amount in the body is only 25 milligrams. Deficiency can develop in a few weeks on low intake. It is probably the quickest vitamin deficiency to develop in people who for any reason have appetite loss or extended episodes of vomiting, or in those who restrict their diets or fast because of obesity.

Whole-grain flours and breads and cereals with bran virtually intact are rich in thiamine, as are liver, lean pork, and fresh green vegetables. But overcooking can destroy much of the vitamin, and thiamine is often lost when stock from meat stews and pot liquor of vegetables are discarded.

Riboflavin (vitamin B_2)

Riboflavin deficiency can produce reduced visual acuity, eye fatigue, oversensitivity to light, itching or watering of the eyes, and seborrheic dermatitis. There are, of course, other causes for these. But when they are the results of riboflavin deficiency, they respond to vitamin supplementation.

And, as the Army study with conscientious objectors indicated, a deficiency of the vitamin can produce depression, hypochondriasis, and other personality changes.

Theoretically, riboflavin deficiency should be rare in the United States. Milk is a good source, but milk exposed to sunlight for three and a half hours can lose up to 75 percent of its riboflavin content. Other good sources include other dairy products and eggs, organ meats, such as liver, kidney, and heart, as well as other meats, poultry, fish, green leafy vegetables, legumes, fruits, and nuts. Sodium bicarbonate used in cooking can destroy the vitamin, and bread fortified with it can lose some riboflavin content on exposure to light.

Need for the vitamin is increased in pregnancy, and a 1971 study found low riboflavin levels occurring often, particularly in the last six weeks of pregnancy.

Niacin (vitamin B_3)

Niacin is involved in many body biochemical reactions, playing an important role in normal functioning of the central nervous system and in maintaining the integrity of the skin and mucous membranes.

As we noted earlier, the ability of a deficiency of niacin to produce the dementia of pellagra stimulated biological psychiatry. By 1955, there were reports of a variety of psychiatric disorders that could, at least sometimės, develop from niacin deficiency and that responded to the vitamin. They included some depressions, delirium, confusional exhaustion, and neurasthenia, or nervous prostration, with fatigue, appetite loss, energy deficiency, and aches and pains.

More recently, niacin has become the subject of considerable controversy in the field of psychiatry as it has been used in massive doses for the treatment of schizophrenia. Some reports have indicated marked improvement in thousands of schizophrenic patients. And there are now many psychiatrists practicing orthomolecular psychiatry, which is based on the belief that schizophrenia and other disturbances are biochemical anomalies rather than genetic, psychogenic, or environmental in nature. In effect, they hold that some people suffer mental and behavioral disturbances because of an inborn difficulty in making proper use of some nutrients, including niacin, and when that is so they respond to doses of nutrients massive enough to make up for the difficulties in handling ordinarily adequate amounts.

Niacin is present in many foods, including fish, organ meats, whole-grain breads and cereals, eggs, milk, poultry, lima beans, and peanuts. But niacin deficiencies occur. They may stem from prolonged diarrheal disease, cirrhosis of the liver, and chronic alcoholism. Simple dietary deficiency—inadequate intake of niacin-rich foods—can occur and is enough of a threat that the Food and Nutrition Board advocated including niacin along with the other nutrients it recommended for increased fortification of foods made of wheat, corn, and rice.

Pyridoxine (vitamin B_6)

First identified in 1934, pyridoxine came into prominence in 1952 when a commercial infant formula caused convulsions and the reason turned out to be that excessive heating during preparation of the formula destroyed pyridoxine. The infants recovered quickly when given injections of the vitamin and no further cases developed when pyridoxine was added to the formula.

Subsequently, a possible relationship between mental retardation and increased need for pyridoxine was indicated when retarded children suffering from convulsions were freed of the convulsions through increased amounts of the vitamin.

There have been reports that some individuals may be pyridoxine-dependent, requiring greater amounts than normal. For example, a study at the Institute for Child Behavior Research in San Diego of eight hundred psychiatric child patients indicated a need for the vitamin ranging from 5 to 400 milligrams a day although the estimated average need in the general population is only about 3.5 milligrams.

Dr. Bernard Rimland of the Institute has used high dosage levels of some vitamins, including pyridoxine, in problem children, with promising results.

Pyridoxine-dependence—a need for larger-than-normal amounts—may sometimes be caused by drugs such as those used for tuberculosis. Oral contraceptives also appear to cause increased need for the vitamin in some users who show mild to moderate depression, irritability, lethargy, and fatigue.

Some men experiencing an anemia that produces lack of energy, easy fatigability, and irritability, sometimes accompanied by vertigo, headache, ear ringing, and spots before the eyes, seem to be pyridoxine-dependent and respond to doses ranging from 50 to 200 milligrams a day.

Special dependency aside, is pyridoxine deficiency common among other people? There have been reports indicating that it is, that the general requirement for about 3½ milligrams a day may be about two and a half times as much as many people ordinarily get.

Pyridoxine occurs in beef liver, kidney, pork loin and ham, leg of veal, fresh fish, bananas, cabbage, avocados, peanuts, walnuts, raisins, prunes, and cereal grains. But vegetables lose some of the vitamin in freezing, and pyridoxine is destroyed by the high temperatures of sterilization for canning. Cereal grains lose up to 90 percent of the vitamin during milling, so commonly used flours and breads and other food products made from such flours almost always are low in pyridoxine.

Cobalamin (vitamin B_{12})

Cobalamin deficiency, as we noted in the earlier chapter on anemia, occurs despite a good intake of the vitamin when an intrinsic factor, needed for absorption and produced by stomach cells, is inadequate or lacking. It can also develop in the presence of an intestinal tapeworm or when certain intestinal bacteria that use the vitamin multiply and consume so much that little is left for the host.

The deficiency can produce such physical symptoms as nausea, abdominal pain, diarrhea, shortness of breath. It can also lead to psychiatric symptoms. There may be memory impairment, dulling of mental awareness and acuity, difficulty in concentration.

When a tapeworm is responsible, the need is for deworming with an anthelmintic agent; when bacteria are the cause, antibiotics may be used. When lack of intrinsic factor is involved, periodic injections of the vitamin eliminate all symptoms.

Folic acid

A deficiency of this B vitamin, as we noted earlier, can lead to fatigue, headaches, constipation, sensations of dizziness, and vision blurring.

In some cases, it may be responsible for weakness, irritability, sleeplessness and forgetfulness, and even depression.

A deficiency can be induced easily enough. Body stores of folic acid are small, about enough to last a month. The vitamin occurs in many plant and animal tissues; richest sources are yeast, liver, and green vegetables; moderate amounts are in dairy foods, meat, and fish.

But folic acid is unstable when exposed to air and to ultraviolet light and declines steadily in storage. Cooking, especially boiling, and the heat preservation in canning can destroy up to 90 percent of it.

Folic acid also may be depleted and folic acid supplementation may be needed when some drugs are used. They include oral contraceptives; phenobarbitone, phenytoin, and primidone, which are used for epilepsy; methotrexate, sometimes used for cancer and severe psoriasis; and pyrimethamine, an antimalarial.

Magnesium

Only recently has the importance of the metal magnesium in the body economy begun to be fully recognized. It's now known to be involved in many of the most basic aspects of body chemistry. It is needed for nerve and muscle activity and, among other things, for the activation of enzyme systems involved in the use of other minerals, vitamins, even proteins, and in producing and transferring energy.

Recent studies have shown magnesium deficiency to be capable of producing many physical disturbances, including abnormal heart rhythms, and twitching and tremors of any and all muscles. It has been reported by some investigators to be sometimes involved in blood vessel disorders such as phlebothrombosis and by other researchers to be sometimes a factor in toxemias of pregnancy.

There have also been recent reports that magnesium deficiency may produce mental symptoms that can range from relatively mild apathy and memory impairment to confusion, disorientation, hallucinations, and paranoia.

At the University of Montreal international conference on magnesium, referred to earlier, Dr. Edmund B. Flick of the West Virginia University Department of Medicine keynoted the research results presented by many investigating teams by emphasizing that the manifestations of magnesium deficiency are many and varied; that the deficiency is common; that, although it is common, it is often undetected.

When, for example, University of Wisconsin investigators made a study of a group of pregnant women, they found that no woman obtained the 450 milligrams a day recommended by the Food and Nutrition Board; 98 percent ingested less than 70 percent of the recommended amount; 79 percent got less than 55 percent of the amount.

At the University of Colorado Hospital, when researchers made a special study to check on magnesium deficiency, they found it in 205, or 14.5 percent, of 1,418 patients, and found, too, that commonly physicians treating the patients had no suspicion of the deficiency and would not have requested a test for it.

Is magnesium deficiency widespread? Nobody really knows, but there is some concern that it may be. For one thing, increased softening of water may be responsible to some extent. Along with calcium, magnesium is what imparts hardness to water, and much of it is removed in the softening process.

Another significant factor could be use of highly refined flour. Minerals as well as vitamins are lost in the heavy milling of fiber, which involves the stripping away of virtually all the mineral- and vitamin-rich bran. And when flour and bread "enrichment" was instituted, no provision was made for adding magnesium.

Zinc

Zinc is another mineral whose multiple importance to the body has only recently become apparent. It is now known to be necessary for growth, sexual maturation, and as a component of many vital enzymes.

One of the first findings was that an oral zinc supplement often could speed up delayed healing of a wound. It appeared that in burns and after surgery, even in some patients with previously adequate body stores of zinc, there might be enough depletion to interfere with healing.

Another striking development came in 1971 when National Institutes of Health investigators found that zinc deficiency often was the cause of lost or perverted senses of taste and smell in patients whose problem had previously been entirely mysterious and frequently had been considered psychogenic. The investigators studied some four thousand people, men and women, aged 25 to 81. All had low blood levels of zinc; all responded to zinc supplements.

Zinc has also been used with good results in promoting growth in undersized people found to have zinc deficiency, both children and adults.

That zinc deficiency may sometimes be responsible for mental changes—poor memory, depression, disorientation—and that these can be overcome by zinc supplementation has been shown in recent work at the Baylor College of Medicine.

Is zinc deficiency common? Some authorities believe it is. One of the pioneer zinc investigators is Dr. Harold H. Sandstead of the U.S. Department of Agriculture Human Nutrition Laboratory, Grand Forks, North Dakota.

Not long ago, in the *American Journal of Clinical Nutrition,* Sandstead observed that "the hypothesis that zinc nutriture of many Americans is marginal would have seemed ridiculous several years ago. Today, this is no longer the case. Advances in knowledge of the metabolic role of zinc, factors which influence its availability for absorption, and the effects of zinc deficiency in man have made it apparent that we must be concerned with the adequacy of the American diet as a source of zinc and with human zinc requirements."

Dr. Richard W. Luecke, a Michigan State University biochemist, has reported that "there is ample reason to suspect that zinc intakes of a number of individuals in this country may be marginal. Zinc shortages can be found in all people, rich or poor."

Total body zinc stores are not large. An average adult male, for example, has 2.2 grams in his 154 pounds of body weight.

Investigators have found that the average American diet contains 8 to 16 milligrams of zinc per day, that the average healthy person needs at least 12 milligrams per day to stay in balance, and that illness or injury increases these requirements.

In the normal person in zinc balance, about 50 percent of the daily intake, or 6 milligrams, is absorbed. Of this, 5 milligrams is secreted back through liver and pancreas products and passes out in the stool and about ½ milligram appears in the urine and another ½ milligram is lost in sweat, cast-off hair, and skin.

Zinc is—or should be—widely distributed in foods. But

the mineral is largely removed from wheat and other grains and from sugar by refining. And there is some concern about growing zinc deficiency in plants. Dr. Frank G. Viets, Jr., of the Department of Agriculture has reported marked increases in crop zinc deficits over the past twenty years and findings of zinc deficiencies in plants in at least thirty states. One troubled prediction is that unless leached-out soil zinc is replaced on a wide scale, more and more people will develop symptoms of zinc deficiency.

The natural zinc content of foods varies considerably. In parts of zinc per million parts of food, the general averages are: seafoods, 17.5; meats, 30.6; dairy products, 8.8; cereals and grains, 17.7; legume vegetables, 10.7; root vegetables, 3.4; leafy vegetables, 1.7; fats and oils, 8.4; nuts, 34.2; fruits, 0.5; beverages, 0.2; condiments, 22.9.

Zinc content also varies greatly within food groups. Fresh oysters, for example, contain 1,487 parts per million; canned tuna, 29.1; canned sardines, 29.1; frozen shrimp, 14.8; frozen lobster, 1.5. Among meats, round steak, with 56.6, and lamb chops, with 55.3, are richest, while ground beef contains 25 ppm; liver, 39.2; pork loin, 18.9; pork chops, 3.6; chicken legs, 29.1. Whole egg contains 20.8; nonfat dry milk, 35.1; homogenized milk, only 0.5 or less. Among condiments, caraway seeds contain 2.8; cinnamon, 13.4; black pepper, 18.3; and ground mustard, 22.9.

Combating nutrition-related behavioral disturbances

Once a nutritional disturbance is suspected as a possible factor in a behavioral problem, its diagnosis may be aided by blood or other tests to determine body levels of a possibly deficient nutrient.

Certainly, there are many other possible causes for behavioral problems.

But there may be grounds for suspicion of nutritional involvement because of the presence of a physical disorder—an ulcer or a problem of malabsorption, for example—

which could be responsible for failure to absorb adequate quantities of one or more nutrients or for inability to properly utilize them.

There may be grounds for suspicion when drugs known to be capable of interfering with utilization of some nutrients or increasing requirements for them are used—oral contraceptives and anticonvulsants, for example.

There may be grounds for suspicion, too, when the diet is limited in amount or in variety for any of many reasons—weight reduction, adherence to fad regimens, chewing difficulties, for example.

When, in fact, a nutritional deficiency is involved, rushing to ingest huge quantities of vitamins or minerals or both is not a panacea.

Is the deficiency the result of a physical problem (such as ulcer or malabsorption) that may not have been previously detected or if detected not adequately treated? Then the physical problem deserves immediate attention.

Is the deficiency related to use of some medication? Then that specific nutrient with which the medication interferes or interacts needs to be supplemented.

And if poor diet is the cause of deficiency, the diet needs attention.

17. *Drug-induced Behavioral Disturbances*

- A middle-aged woman suddenly experiences great restlessness, weakness, appetite loss, and burning and tingling sensations. The cause turns out to be a drug, Hydrodiuril, taken for edema.
- A young man first becomes increasingly nervous, then confused, and goes on to hallucinate. The reason: an antihistamine drug, Periactin, taken for allergy.
- A successful businessman suddenly finds himself extremely anxious for no reason he can think of. The cause: a drug, Rauzide, taken for high blood pressure.
- A woman who begins to experience dizziness, excitability, and speech slurring is quickly relieved when a drug, Equanil, being used for anxiety is stopped.

Almost all blessings can be mixed and those of medicine are no exceptions. Although therapeutic drugs have made significant contributions to health and welfare, none is without potential side effect.

Antibiotics obviously have been lifesavers. But if penicillin can cure pneumonia, it can sometimes produce allergic reactions, even potentially lethal ones. Other antibiotics, such as the "mycins," cutting a wide swath among intestinal fauna, may sometimes decimate beneficial bacterial populations, allowing hardier and previously minority strains to multiply and cause digestive upsets.

A possibility of emotional and behavioral upsets from therapeutic drugs? Indeed. And even from drugs meant to calm and soothe.

One of the most serious adverse effects of major tranquilizers is called tardive dyskinesia: grotesque facial distortions, protrusion of the tongue, lower jaw tics, other involuntary mouth-area movements. The most frequent adverse reaction of major tranquilizers, akathisia, consists of great internal daytime restlessness, especially of the legs, and a compulsion to move, with the restlessness sometimes extending to painful restless insomnia at night.

Many drugs for many purposes—sedatives, minor tranquilizers, antidepressants, pain relievers, heart drugs, hormones, and still others—can on occasion produce mental and behavioral symptoms as well as physical side effects.

The incidence of drug-related psychiatric side effects is not huge, but neither is it insignificant. One collaborative drug surveillance program found a 2.8 percent incidence.

"Drug-induced symptoms," a recent medical report warns, "are among the most frequent causes of sudden-onset emotional reactions, and all practicing physicians should be aware of the potential when prescribing drugs or treating a patient who may already be taking medication for a preexisting condition."

Should patients know about the potential, however small, of a prescribed drug for causing trouble? Some physicians still think not, believing that such knowledge will only cause needless anxiety. More and more others, however, believe that a well-informed patient is a protected patient.

Early recognition by a patient of a possible association of a new symptom or set of symptoms with a medication being used can save needless worry, anxiety, and suffering. All that may be needed to minimize or eliminate the undesirable effects may be a change in dosage. Failing that, it is very often possible to change medication, using another that, for a particular patient, can be effective without penalty.

In the pages that follow, you'll find information on the more commonly used drugs of many kinds and the psychiatric as well as other disturbances they may cause.

It is important to emphasize again that such disturbances are the exceptions rather than the rule, and that when a medication is necessary, when it has been properly prescribed, the risk is worth the benefit, and the risk can be greatly minimized or even eliminated by prompt action of the patient, and then of the physician, should there be any untoward development.

Major tranquilizers

These are drugs, also known as neuroleptics, used for serious psychiatric problems such as schizophrenia, and some of them, sometimes, for other purposes such as to control severe nausea and vomiting, to relieve excessive anxiety, tension, and agitation associated with serious physical illness, and for overcoming otherwise unyielding hiccups.

The major tranquilizers include Compazine, Etrafon, Haldol, Mellaril, Navane, Prolixin, Serentil, Stelazine, Taractan, Thorazine, Tindal, Triavil, and Trilafon.

As already noted above, one of the more serious adverse effects is tardive dyskinesia and one of the most frequent is akathisia.

Other possible emotional/behavioral disturbances: agitation, anxiety, depression, drowsiness, confusion, lethargy, euphoria, grand mal seizures, hallucinations, jitteriness.

Possible physical disturbances include blood disorders, jaundice, racing heartbeat, breast engorgement, vision disturbances, menstrual irregularities, impotence, skin outbreaks, headache, insomnia, swallowing difficulty, constipation, diarrhea, nausea, vomiting.

Minor tranquilizers

These are drugs commonly used for tension and anxiety.

Among preparations that are minor tranquilizers or contain them as ingredients are Atarax, Deprol, Equanil, Librax, Libritabs, Librium, Menrium, Meprospan, Miltown, Miltrate, Pathibamate, Raudixin, Rau-Sed, Sandril, Serpasil, Valium, and Vistaril.

They may sometimes produce as adverse reactions any or several such emotional/behavioral disturbances as drowsiness, slurred speech, weakness, euphoria, overstimulation, paradoxical excitement, incoordination. Some may cause depression, nervousness, paradoxical anxiety, nightmares.

Other adverse effects that may occur include nausea, vomiting, appetite loss, diarrhea, nasal congestion, itching, rash, impotence, decreased libido, muscle aches, vision disturbances, chills, anemia.

Antidepressants

These are drugs used to relieve the symptoms of mental depression.

They include Adapin, Aventyl, Deprol, Elavil, Endep, Etrafon, Imavate, imipramine hydrochloride, Janimine, Marplan, Nardil, Norpramin, Parnate, Pertofrane, Presamine, Sinequan, SK-Pramine, Tofranil, Triavil, and Vivactil.

They may sometimes produce as adverse reactions such disturbances as confusional states, disturbed concentration, disorientation, delusions, hallucinations, excitement, anxiety, restlessness, insomnia, nightmares, numbness or tingling sensations, incoordination, tremors, seizures.

Other adverse effects that may occur include dry mouth, vision disturbances, skin rash, hives, racing pulse, palpitation, heart rhythm disturbance, nausea, vomiting, appetite loss, peculiar taste, diarrhea, blacktongue, testicular and breast swelling in men, dizziness, weakness, fatigue, headache, weight gain or loss, drowsiness, hair loss.

Antihypertensives

These are drugs used to reduce elevated blood pressure. Some also have a diuretic action that helps to eliminate excess fluids from the body and may be used for other conditions such as congestive heart failure in which there is abnormal fluid accumulation.

Antihypertensive compounds include Aldactazide, Aldactone, Aldoclor, Aldomet, Aldoril, Apresazide, Apresoline, Butaserpazide, Catapres, Combipres, Diucardin, Diupres, Diuril, Diutensen, Dyazide, Enduron, Enduronyl, Esidrix, Esimil, Eutonyl, Eutron, Exna, Harmonyl, HydroDiuril, Hydromox, Hydropres, Hydrotensin, Hygroton, Inderal, Ismelin, Metahydrin, Metatensin, Minipres, Moderil, Naqua, Naquival, Naturetin, Nipride, Oretic, Oreticyl, Raudixin, Rau-Sed, Rauzide, Regroton, Renese, Saluron, Salutensin, Ser-Ap-Es, Serpasil, Singoserp-Esidrix, SK-Reserpine, Unipres, and Unitensen.

Not all have exactly the same side effects, but drugs in this class may occasionally produce such adverse reactions as sedation, weakness, light-headedness, decreased mental acuity, depression, other psychic disturbances, including nightmares and reversible mild psychoses, incoordination, lethargy, restlessness.

Other possible adverse reactions include anemia, appetite loss, blood disturbances, cramps, diarrhea, fever, headache, hives, itching, impotence, jaundice, abnormal hair growth, rash, nausea, vomiting.

Antihistamines

These are drugs that may be used to relieve hay fever and other allergies, symptoms of the common cold, motion sickness, and for other purposes.

Antihistamine preparations include Actidil, Actifed, Allerest, Ambenyl, Benadryl, Chlor-Trimeton, Citra, Citra Forte, Codimal, Co-Pyronil, Coricidin, Coriforte, Corilin,

Deconamine, Demazin, Dimetane, Dimetapp, Disomer, Disophrol, Dramamine, Drinus, Drixoral, Duadacin, Emesert, Extendryl, Fedahist, Fedrazil, Fiogesic, Forhistal, Hispril, Histabid, Histadyl, Histaspan, Historal, Isoclor, Kronohist, Marhist, Matropinal, Napril, Narine, Neotep, Nolamine, Oraminic, PBZ-SR, Periactin, Phenergan, Polaramine, Pyribenzamine, Quelidrine, Rhinex, Rondec, Rynatan, Rynatuss, Sinovan, Sinulin, SK-Diphenhydramine, Stopp, Tacaryl, Teldrin, Triaminic, Triaminicin, Triten, Tussagesic, Ursinus, Vistaril, and ZiPan.

These agents may sometimes produce any or several such disturbances as drowsiness, confusion, nervousness, restlessness, insomnia, excitement, fatigue.

Other possible adverse reactions include nausea, vomiting, diarrhea, vision disturbances, difficulty in urination, constipation, nasal stuffiness, chest tightness and wheezing, vertigo, palpitation, headache, insomnia, hives, rash, dryness of mouth, nose, and throat, tingling, heaving, and weakness of hands.

Antispasmodics and anticholinergics

These drugs are often used for peptic ulcer, irritable bowel, and other spasmodic and colicky conditions of the gastrointestinal tract and urinary tract.

They include Anaspaz, Antrenyl, Antrocol, Arco-Lase, atropine sulfate, Barbidonna, Bar-Tropin, Belap, Belladenal, Bentyl, Cantil, Chardonna, Combid, Cytospaz, Darbid, Daricon, Ditropan, Dolonil, Donnatal, Donphen, Dranochol, Dynspas, Enarax, Eta-Lent, Festalan, Gustase, Hepahydrin, Homapin, Hybephen, Kinesed, Kutrase, Levsin/Phenobarbital, Levsinex, Librax, Matropinal, Milpath, Octin, Pamine Bromide, papaverine, Pathibamate, Pathilon, Prantal, Pro-Banthine, Probital, Prydon, Quarzan, Robinul, Sedadrops, Sed-Tens, Sidonna, Trac, Tral, Trasentine, Trest, Trocinate, Uretron, Urised, Urispas, Valpin, and Vistrax.

Such agents may sometimes produce any or several such

disturbances as mental confusion or excitement, drowsiness, insomnia, nervousness.

Other possible adverse reactions include constipation, bloated feeling, dizziness, headache, hives, impotence, mouth dryness, taste loss, nausea, vomiting, palpitation, fast pulse, vision disturbances, decreased sweating, urinary hesitancy, urinary retention.

Anti-inflammatory agents

These drugs are used for a wide variety of problems, including severe allergies, asthma, arthritic and rheumatic disorders, kidney conditions, and blood disorders.

Among preparations that are anti-inflammatory agents or contain them as ingredients are Aristocort, Arthropan, Azolid, Betapar, Butazolidin, Celestone, Cortenema, Cortisporin, Decaderm in Estergel, Decadron, Dermacort, Deronil, Dexone, Diprosone, Fluonid, Flurobate, Halog, Hysone, Kenacort, Kenalog, Lidex, Locorten, Medrol, Meticortelone, Meticorten, Metreton, Motrin, Nalfon, Naprosyn, Orabase, Orasone, Plaquenil, Proctocort, SK-Prednisone, SK-Triamcinolone, Sterane, Sterazolidin, Synalar, and Tolectin.

Some of these agents may sometimes produce such disturbances as agitation, confusion, irritability.

Other possible adverse reactions include fluid retention, muscle weakness, peptic ulcer, abdominal distention, vertigo, headache, menstrual irregularities, anemia, facial redness, fractures, dizziness, thin, fragile skin, diarrhea, blood disturbances, fever, joint pain, vision blurring, nausea, vomiting, insomnia, lethargy.

Anticonvulsants

These are drugs used for the control of various types of epileptic seizures.

Anticonvulsants include Celontin, Clonopin, Dilantin,

Gemonil, Mebaral, Mesantoin, Milontin, Mysoline, Paradione, Peganone, Phelantin, Phenurone, Tegretol, Tridione, Valium, and Zarontin.

Drugs of this class may sometimes produce such disturbances as drowsiness, incoordination, confusion, fatigue, hallucinations, speech disturbances, depression with agitation, talkativeness, irritability, nervousness.

Other possible adverse reactions include anemia, blood disturbances, skin rashes, nausea, vomiting, jaundice, hair loss, weight gain, diarrhea, abdominal pain, constipation, hiccups, headache, vision blurring, insomnia.

Sedatives

These are drugs that may be used to sedate or calm nervousness, irritability, and excitement, and as hypnotics to help induce sleep.

They include Allurate, Amytal, Arco-Lase Plus, Belap, Buticaps, Butisol Sodium, Cantil/Phenobarbital, Carbrital, Dialog, Dolatrin, Donphen, Emesert, Eskabarb, Gustase Plus, Levsin/Phenobarbital, Levsinex/Phenobarbital, Matropinal, Mebaral, Nembutal, Oxoids, Pamine, Plexonal, Repan, S.B.P. Plus, Seconal, Sedadrops, Sedapap, Sed-Tens Ty-Med, SK-Phenobarbital, Solfoton, and Tuinal, all of which belong to the barbiturate family. Others, nonbarbiturates, include Aquachloral, Beta-Chlor, Bromural, Dalmane, Equanil, Levoprome, Noctec, Noludar, Parest, Phenergan, Quaalude, SK-Chloral Hydrate, Sopor, Tranxene, and ZiPan.

Such drugs may sometimes produce such disturbances as confusion, drowsiness, lethargy, paradoxical excitement, light-headedness, staggering, depression, euphoria, disorientation, nervousness, apprehension, speech slurring.

Other possible adverse reactions may include headache, heartburn, upset stomach, nausea, vomiting, diarrhea, chest pain, body and joint pain, skin rash, itching, dry mouth, shortness of breath, faintness.

Antianginal drugs

These are drugs used to relieve or prevent the chest pain, angina pectoris, associated with coronary heart disease.

They include amyl nitrite, Antora, Duotrate, Inderal, Iso-Bid, Isordil, Miltrate, Nitrobid, Nitroglyn, Nitrong, Nitrostat, Papavatral, papaverine, Paveril, Peritrate, Persantine, SK-Petn, sorbide, and Sorbitrate.

Occasionally some of these agents may produce such disturbances as mental depression (manifested by insomnia, lassitude, weakness, and fatigue), hallucinations, short-term memory loss, emotional lability, overstimulation, excitement.

Other possible adverse reactions may include nausea, vomiting, abdominal cramping, diarrhea, constipation, rash, flushing, headache, pallor, excessive sweating.

Antiarrhythmic drugs

These are drugs used to correct various types of abnormal heart rhythms.

They include Cardioquin, Inderal, Isuprel, ouabain, Pronestyl, quinidine, Quinora, and SK-Quinidine.

Occasionally such agents may cause such disturbances as depression, fatigue, hallucinations, giddiness, apprehension, confusion, excitement.

Other possible adverse reactions include breathing difficulty, dizziness, gastrointestinal upset, fever, headache, hearing disturbance, rash, cold sweat, vision disturbance, hives, itching, bitter taste.

Digitalis preparations for the heart

These are drugs that have a tonic effect on the heart and are among the most valued of medications for certain heart conditions, including congestive heart failure and some abnormal rhythms.

Digitalis preparations include Acylanid, Cedilanid, Crystodigin, digoxin, Gitaligin, Lanoxin, and SK-Digoxin.

Adjusting the dose for the individual patient to achieve the beneficial effects of these preparations without the undesirable effects that can come from overdosage is one of the fine arts of medicine.

With overdosage, there may be any of such disturbances as apathy, weakness, headache, visual disturbances, appetite loss, nausea, vomiting, diarrhea, premature beats and other heart rhythm disturbances.

Oral contraceptives

These hormonal preparations designed to prevent pregnancy include Brevicon, Demulen, Enovid, Loestrin, Lo/Ovral, Micronor, Modicon, No-Q.D., Norinyl, Norlestrin, Ortho-Novum, Ovral, Ovrette, Ovulen, and Zorane.

The oral contraceptives may sometimes produce such disturbances as depression, fatigue, nervousness, libido change.

Other possible adverse effects include abdominal bloating and cramps, backache, breast tenderness, breast enlargement, breast secretion, blood pressure rise, symptoms similar to those of bladder infection, edema, eye neuritis, dizziness, hirsutism, itching, jaundice, migraine, nausea, vomiting, pulmonary embolism, rash, retinal thrombosis, scalp hair loss, stroke, thrombophlebitis, skin pigmentation, weight change.

Sulfonamides for infection

These antibacterial drugs are useful for many types of infection, including some that do not yield readily to antibiotics. Some also are useful for other purposes such as in the treatment of ulcerative colitis.

The sulfonamides include Azulfidine, Bactrim, Gantanol, Gantrisin, Midicel, Renoquid, Sebizon, Septra, SK-Soxazole, Sulfa, Sulfamylon, Terfonyl, and Thiosulfil.

Occasionally the drugs may produce such adverse reactions as apathy, fatigue, mental depression, nervousness, hallucinations.

Other possible adverse effects include headache, nausea, vomiting, abdominal pains, diarrhea, anemias, skin eruptions, joint pains, chills, fever.

Anti-Parkinsonism drugs

These agents, useful for helping to control Parkinsonism, or shaking palsy, include Akineton, Artane, Bendopa, Cogentin, Disipal, Dopar, Kemadrin, Larodopa, Levsin, Levsinex, Pagitane, Sinemet, Symmetrel, and Tremin.

Occasionally these drugs may produce such disturbances as depression, disorientation, euphoria, anxiety, irritability, confusion, hallucinations, nervousness, agitation.

Other adverse reactions may include appetite loss, nausea, headache, dry mouth, sense of weakness, fatigue, vision blurring, skin rash, numbness of fingers, constipation.

18. And More: The Growing Somatopsychic Catalog

Psychosomatic medicine is really a broad concept. It is meant to be concerned with the study of the interrelationships of psyche and soma.

Certainly, mind can influence body—and often does. It can do so to the extent of triggering or exacerbating physical illness.

Psychosomatic medicine is meant to encompass not only this but the reverse—the capacity of physical malfunction to produce emotional illness and behavioral disturbances. The use of "somatopsychic"—a term turnaround to emphasize body over mind—is beginning to have increasing currency.

Beyond those mentioned earlier in this book, other problems—previously not thought of in terms of physical origins or, in some cases, sometimes but not often enough thought of—are being described.

A new link: dementia and high blood fat levels

The woman was one of a small group of patients with mystifying symptoms seen at the Baylor College of Medicine Department of Neurology in Houston. She was 57 and until two years before had been a successful real-estate agent. At that point, however, she had begun to suffer from irritability, depression, anxiety, episodes of crying without reason, and failing memory. Subsequently, she developed other symptoms—dizzy spells, lack of coordination, tingling and numbness in both feet and occasionally in her fingers and hands.

She received thorough study for diabetes, cirrhosis of the liver, hypothyroidism, pancreatitis, and other disorders that conceivably might be responsible. She had none of these. But there was one remarkable physical finding: grossly elevated blood fat levels—cholesterol at 600 and triglycerides at 1,600.

It took a combination of diet and a medication, clofibrate, to lower those levels. Over a three-month period, cholesterol came down to 217 and triglycerides to 183. At that point, all her symptoms disappeared.

In five other patients seen at Baylor, similar symptoms—a kind of hyperlipidemic (high blood fat level) dementia—responded to diet alone to bring down the excessive levels.

The mechanism by which the excessive levels can produce the neuropathies, or nervous system problems, is unknown. "But the fact that patients improve when their hyperlipidemia is treated," report the Baylor neurologists, "makes it desirable to look for this defect in all patients with dementia and treat it as soon as it's found."

Fatigue, headache, fainting and smoker's polycythemia

Polycythemia is a blood disorder quite the opposite of anemia. Instead of too few red blood cells, there are too many, so much so that the increased thickening of the blood and increased viscosity impair flow.

The symptoms may include fatigability, decreased efficiency, difficulty in concentration, headache, drowsiness, forgetfulness, and fainting, all the results of diminished supply of blood to the brain and other tissues.

The symptoms are the same no matter what the form of

polycythemia—and there are two basic forms. In one, called polycythemia vera, for reasons not understood, there is overgrowth of the blood-cell-forming tissues of the bone marrow.

In the other basic form, called secondary polycythemia, oxygen supply to the tissues is decreased and the body attempts to compensate by making more red blood cells. Living at high altitude can produce polycythemia, as can severe chronic lung and heart disorders.

Recently, evidence that excessive smoking can cause polycythemia has come from a number of studies. One of the more striking was made by Drs. J. Robert Smith and Stephen A. Landaw of the Veterans Administration Hospital and the State University of New York-Upstate Medical Center, Syracuse, with twenty-two patients—eighteen men and four women—all excessive cigar or cigarette smokers and all with polycythemia.

Three of the patients stopped smoking entirely and two others markedly reduced their smoking. In all five, red blood cell volumes returned to normal and symptoms disappeared within several days. In the other patients, symptoms continued as long as they continued to smoke.

Why should smoking provoke polycythemia? There are high levels of carbon monoxide in tobacco smoke. The carbon monoxide inhaled has a strong affinity, or attachment, for hemoglobin, the red cell pigment that picks up oxygen from the lungs and carries it to tissues. The carbon monoxide replaces the oxygen, leads to tissue oxygen shortage, and to the efforts by the body to compensate by increasing red blood cell production.

"Considering the wide use of tobacco," Drs. Smith and Landaw reported recently in the *New England Journal of Medicine*, "smoking should be one of the largest single causes of polycythemia."

FMF and fever, pain, depression

FMF is a disorder of unknown cause. Its full name—familial Mediterranean fever—is a misnomer. And until recently, it has often defied even the best diagnosticians and virtually all treatments.

On the average, a victim experiences an attack every two to four weeks, each lasting one to three days. FMF can produce fever of unknown origin, or severe abdominal pain, or both. Few patients escape at least one exploratory abdominal operation that reveals nothing. Severe depression, addiction to drugs, underachievement, and interference with careers are common consequences.

A breakthrough finally came just a few years ago when a 23-year-old woman with FMF was admitted to Massachusetts General Hospital in Boston in coma after having become so depressed that she had swallowed eighty pentobarbital tablets.

Like many other FMF victims, she had been experiencing attacks of fever and severe abdominal pain for many years. She had previously undergone abdominal surgery, including removal of her gall bladder without results. A low-fat diet, cortisonelike drugs, psychotherapy, and still other treatments had all been tried, but nothing seemed able to relieve the intensity of her attacks or reduce their frequency.

Today, she is completely free of the disabling pain and fever, working, leading a normal life, thanks to treatment with an old drug, colchicine, long used for gout.

Colchicine was tried in a desperate effort to help the young woman, who remained in coma for four days after taking the barbiturate. Seeking advice from many physicians about whether any therapy had ever worked for FMF, Dr. Stephen Goldfinger, the Massachusetts General Hospital gastroenterologist in charge of her case, got only one glimmering of hope. Two Harvard Medical School physicians had started one patient on a trial with one tablet of colchicine twice a day a few years before and he had remained free of attacks as long as he took the medication.

As soon as she was out of coma, the young woman was placed on colchicine three times a day. She stayed free of attacks for two years, and when three attacks then occurred, the medication was increased to four times a day. She has been well ever since.

Goldfinger soon was treating ten other patients with FMF. Through months of colchicine therapy during which there should have been 355 attacks if previous attack frequency prevailed, there were only 7 attacks. Three of the seven occurred shortly after the drug was temporarily discontinued. The four other patients who noted mild pre-attack symptoms of abdominal discomfort found they could prevent full-blown attacks simply by taking an extra colchicine tablet.

"All patients reported dramatic improvement in their life styles," Dr. Goldfinger has reported, with jobs becoming possible for three previously unable to hold them because of the frequency and severity of their attacks.

Very quickly, confirmation of colchicine's value in FMF came from trials by the National Institute of Allergy and Infectious Diseases and from others abroad.

How colchicine works in FMF is not clear. But Goldfinger sees another value for it as well: as a diagnostic aid. FMF is difficult to diagnose, and the name itself doesn't help, although it sticks despite the fact the disease does not necessarily follow a familial pattern. It can strike an individual without any family history of FMF. Moreover, it is not limited to people of Mediterranean origin but occurs in others as well.

Because of the striking benefit from use of colchicine, suggests Goldfinger, it warrants use as a "diagnostic trial in all patients with recurrent unexplained abdominal pain and fever."

When lupus seems a psychological matter

After attending a college picnic, a 20-year-old girl broke out in a red skin rash over her nose, forehead, and cheeks, shaped somewhat like a butterfly. She had no history of allergy and there was no indication she had come in contact with anything at the picnic that could have caused the rash. It disappeared.

Over the next several years, however, she had more episodes of skin rash, plus attacks of joint pains, fever, pleurisy, and swelling of the feet. Eventually, when protein was found in her urine, a thorough study of her kidneys was made and revealed damage associated with systemic lupus erythematosus (SLE).

SLE, or lupus, as it is also known, is one of the most prominent of what are called autoimmune diseases, those in which the body's defensive immune system produces antibodies that combat no foreign invaders but rather the body's own tissues. In effect, people with autoimmune disease develop allergy to parts of their own bodies.

First noted in young women, SLE is now known to occur in both sexes and to take varied forms. Apparently, in susceptible people, sunlight or latent viral infection can lead to change and leakage of DNA, the genetic material in all cells. Ordinarily, DNA is confined to the nuclei of cells. When it leaks out, getting into the circulation, the immune system responds, producing antibodies to the material.

The outlook for SLE today is good when the disease is diagnosed and properly treated. It is for the young woman, who has responded to medical management with total remission and who is today planning marriage and a family. Dreaded only a few years ago, almost all cases of lupus can now be controlled, if not cured.

But the problem can lie in diagnosis.

One of the principal SLE investigative programs currently under way in the United States is under the direction of Dr. Ronald I. Carr at the National Jewish Hospital and Research Center, Denver.

Carr says SLE is sometimes called "the great impostor" because it so often resembles and is frequently diagnosed as any number of other ailments.

Common symptoms of SLE are a rash, weakness and lack of energy, diminished appetite and weight loss, chronic low-grade fever, and frequent infections. Unless a physician is alert to the possibilities of SLE, such symptoms may not suggest it.

To complicate matters, SLE can affect various systems of the body. It can attack the nervous system, and in so doing may sometimes produce convulsions as the first manifestation, suggesting epilepsy. Or, when it affects the nervous system, it may produce mental disturbances that may make the victim appear to be neurotic or even schizophrenic. In the abdomen, it may seem to be ulcers. If it attacks the joints, it may be mistaken for rheumatoid arthritis or rheumatic fever.

Some patients suffer spasms of the small blood vessels in the fingertips and toes, often following exposure to cold or after some emotional stimulation, and the skin sometimes blanches (Raynaud's phenomenon). Easy bruising also may occur. Another of the strange manifestations of SLE is the occurrence of a false positive test for syphilis, a situation that has created needless grief for many prospective brides and grooms and their families. (There is no known relationship between SLE and any venereal disease, and further testing of those with indicated syphilis can easily determine whether venereal disease is present and may identify the real culprit as SLE.)

Another of the problems with SLE, increasing the difficulty in diagnosis, is that manifestations can come and go spontaneously and may vary sharply in a short period of time. Many patients who have suffered SLE for years have been thought by their physicians to have a problem that is purely psychological.

SLE is now known to be far more common than was ever before imagined. The Kaiser Foundation in San Francisco recently tested all 120,000 of its patients, the largest mass testing program for SLE in history. The results surprised most of the researchers: the incidence of SLE was 1 person out of every 2,000, which would make the disease more common than muscular dystrophy, multiple sclerosis, or leukemia.

The Kaiser Foundation tests and others indicate that SLE is at least five times more common among women than men. It has been diagnosed in people as young as 2 years and as old as 97, most often in women between the ages of 15 and 30.

There may be an inherited susceptibility to the disease. Fairly commonly, a history of related diseases, such as rheumatoid arthritis, in which there are immunologic abnormalities, is found in families of SLE patients. More than one case of SLE may occur in a family but this is unusual.

Blood tests can be helpful in the diagnosis of SLE.

The disease now is considered neither fatal on the one hand nor curable on the other, although occasional deaths are attributed to it and some people eventually show complete regression of all symptoms. Nine out of ten patients with SLE now live ten years or longer; in medical terms, survival for ten years with a disease means an excellent projected outlook for an essentially normal life span.

Good treatment is individualized, depending upon the location and severity of the disease. Among the drugs that may be used singly or in combination are aspirin and aspirinlike compounds, chloroquine or a similar agent, and a cortisonelike drug such as prednisone.

Personality change and the copper disorder

Among the patients seen at Boston's Beth Israel Hospital not long ago was a 12-year-old girl who had been considered schizophrenic because of her peculiar facial expressions and body movements and her failure to speak. But a blood test revealed Wilson's disease, a heritable disorder in the body's handling of copper.

Copper is an essential mineral in small amounts and is obtained by the body in the diet. But in Wilson's disease, copper absorption is accelerated, and an affected individual has, from birth, more copper in the body than is needed.

Early in the disease, there are no symptoms of any kind. But as copper progressively accumulates in various tissues, symptoms develop. When some of the red blood cells take up copper, anemia may occur. In some patients, the liver may be affected and there may be cirrhosis and edema, or waterlogging, of body tissues. In some cases, kidney function is affected.

Copper sometimes may accumulate in the brain. The disease then can be manifested in personality changes that can progress even to dementia, and other symptoms may include tremors, difficulty in speaking, drooling, incoordination, open-mouthedness, and rigidity.

The untreated disease is fatal. Treatment, however, can be effective. It may include use of a drug, penicillamine, which has the ability to chelate, or latch, onto copper and cause it to be excreted. Dietary measures are valuable and are directed at preventing further copper accumulation by avoidance of foods high in copper, such as organ meats, shellfish, nuts, dried legumes, chocolate, and whole-grain cereals.

Queer spells and hyperventilation

One of the most occult, neglected, underdiagnosed syndromes in all of medicine is hyperventilation, or overbreathing, which can be responsible for a wide array of symptoms. So reported Dr. Herbert E. Walker of New York University School of Medicine, New York City, at a recent annual meeting of the American Psychiatric Association.

In more than one hundred patients with phobic, or abnormal, fear and other panic attacks, Walker found, hyperventilation always played a significant role yet was seldom diagnosed. Hyperventilation, he also noted, may lead to such other symptoms as feelings of impending disaster, light-headedness, scalp and neck tightness, tingling and burning sensations, chest pain, and palpitations.

The Walker report was the latest of many.

In hyperventilation, breathing may be abnormally prolonged and deep. The overbreathing isn't necessarily apparent to the individual involved or to onlookers. Because of the excessive breathing, there is an abnormally large loss of carbon dioxide in the expired air, which results in a biochemical disturbance called respiratory alkalosis.

In addition to the symptoms mentioned by Walker, the alkalosis can lead to others: faintness, spells of dizziness and sometimes even blacking out, smothering sensations, throat fullness, pain over the stomach region.

Hyperventilation can be caused by emotional stress and can then go on to add greatly to the stress.

Whether or not hyperventilation is responsible for alarming symptoms often can be determined simply by having a patient deliberately overbreathe, whereupon the typical symptoms for that patient will be reproduced.

Often, an attack of symptoms caused by hyperventilation can be relieved quickly by rebreathing in a paper bag to replace the carbon dioxide that has been blown off.

Dr. Walker has reported that a simple technique of breathing slowly through the nose with the mouth closed will often end or avert an attack.

Recently, too, a British study with seven hundred patients with hyperventilation symptoms at Papworth and Addenbrookes Hospital, Cambridge, indicates that basic to hyperventilation is a poor breathing habit that can permit any physical or emotional disturbance to trigger a chain reaction of increased excess breathing. Treatment, Dr. L. C. Lum, director of the study, has reported, starts with first making the patient aware of how symptoms result from hyperventilation (by deliberate overbreathing to reproduce the symptoms), then converting to a slow, diaphragmatic type of breathing, emphasizing use of abdominal muscles and diaphragm. In most patients, once such breathing was adopted, hyperventilation and its symptoms were completely relieved.

Grunting, blinking, shaking, cursing: the strange, misdiagnosed tic syndrome

It begins in childhood or adolescence. It's often misdiagnosed because of symptoms attributed to personality or behavior disorders. One recent study found that the mean length of time between its onset and diagnosis was 11.7 years.

Gilles de la Tourette's syndrome, named after the physician who first described it, is an unusual tic condition. It produces many tics—many of them physical, many of them verbal.

The first symptom may be eye blinking—frequent, repetitive, and rapid. The blinking tic may soon be replaced or accompanied by tics of the neck, trunk, and limbs. In most cases, there are multiple tics; occasionally only one area of the body is involved.

There are also verbal tics, noises or vocalizations that are added to the involuntary movements or that may replace one or more movement tics. The vocalizations include grunting, throat clearing, shouting, barking.

The verbal tics may take the form of coprolalia, or involuntary use of obscene words. Echo phenomena sometimes may occur and include repeating words of others, repeating one's own words, repeating sounds, and imitating movements.

Other symptoms such as repetitive thoughts and movements or obsessions and compulsions can also occur.

More males than females are affected, the ratio running 3 or 4 to 1. And Tourette victims come from all ethnic and religious groups.

In one recent study, Dr. Gerald S. Golden of Albert Einstein College of Medicine, The Bronx, New York, found that diagnosis is delayed when physicians mistake symptoms for transient childhood tics; when they fail to observe abnormal vocalizations during examination; when they misinterpret coughing, throat clearing, and sniffing; when they refer patients to psychiatrists without strong evidence of personality or behavioral disorders.

Another investigator who has studied the Tourette syndrome extensively, Dr. Arthur K. Shapiro of The New York Hospital-Cornell University Medical College, New York City, notes that many physicians feel that the symptoms are an expression of underlying psychological problems, that patients have difficulty asserting themselves and cannot release their anger. But he also emphasizes: "Studies have shown that although some patients may have this conflict, most do not. Even in those where a psychologic problem has been identified, it may be secondary to coping with this syndrome."

One of Shapiro's patients was a 46-year-old married man. His first symptom, eye blinking, began at age 13. Shaking of the head began at 14. At 15, a physician said he had a bad habit and should snap out of it. Several months later, the first involuntary sounds appeared in the form of "heh, heh, heh, hah, hah, hah." A chiropractor then diagnosed an extra set of nerves at the base of his spine and treated him for six months unsuccessfully. At 19, a psychiatrist was consulted and recommended psychotherapy.

Soon after, he was inducted into the Army, but his symptoms became worse and he was discharged with a diagnosis of psychoneurosis. Symptoms progressed and now included severe tics of the head, neck, and shoulder, followed by repeated throat clearing and "heh, heh, heh, hah, hah, hah." He married at age 27 and thereafter his symptoms became more severe. He began to make spitting sounds and movements, repeatedly struck his forehead with his hand or a kitchen utensil.

He sought help from Veterans Administration as well as private physicians and psychiatrists. He was treated with a variety of suggestive, persuasive, and supportive psychotherapies, hypnosis, an assortment of vitamin, liver, sedative and other drugs. Insulin coma and electroconvulsive treatments were tried without avail.

At age 36, later than its start in most cases, involuntary use of obscene words began. The first words were "cunt, prick, fuck," followed by "son of a bitch, cocksucker, and mother-fucker."

Finally, at age 37, at Johns Hopkins Hospital in Baltimore, the diagnosis of Gilles de la Tourette syndrome was made. Another round of treatment began: shock for three months, insulin coma, psychotherapy, tranquilizers—all ineffective.

It was at age 46, after symptoms had worsened and brain surgery—lobotomy—had been suggested, that the patient received at New York Hospital treatment with haloperidol, then a new investigational drug.

At eleven days after beginning treatment, facial tics, coughing, spitting, barking, and cursing decreased markedly. After four months, the only symptom was one tic every three to four days.

Today, thanks to haloperidol, Tourette syndrome has become treatable, making its early diagnosis all the more important.

Confusion and more from phosphorus deficiency

Phosphorus is a critical constituent of all body tissues, essential for muscle, nervous system, and red blood cell functioning.

Only recently have two things become apparent: the varied situations under which there may be a deficiency of phosphorus and the varied symptoms the deficiency can produce.

Lack of adequate phosphorus can cause muscle weakness, joint stiffness, aching bone pain. It can lead to swallowing difficulty and appetite loss, shallow breathing, tremors, and vertigo. And it can produce memory loss, decreased attention span, confusion, disorientation, and seizures.

Writing recently in *Hospital Practice,* Dr. Robert A. Kreisberg, dean of the College of Medicine at the University of South Alabama, Mobile, reported that, except for the absence of hallucinations, phosphorus deficiency signs and symptoms "can mimic those observed in almost every important neurologic and psychiatric disorder."

Phosphorus deficiency can occur, as might be expected, from severe chronic malnutrition. But it can also occur with prolonged vomiting or severe diarrhea, or when there is a kidney problem that allows large amounts of phosphorus to be lost in the urine.

The deficiency can also develop when, for any reason such as celiac disease or sprue, there is intestinal malabsorption or when there is vitamin D deficiency, which can both decrease phosphorus absorption and increase its excretion. A complication of poorly controlled diabetes, ketoacidosis, can lead to phosphorus deficiency by increasing its loss in the urine.

Alcoholism can produce the deficiency. And so can chronic use of antacids. Most antacids bind phosphate in the gut and prevent its absorption.

Phosphorus depletion deserves consideration in patients showing symptoms the depletion is capable of producing, especially in the presence of conditions—malabsorption, alcoholism, high antacid intake, and others—now known to foster the deficiency.

Blood measurements will indicate whether phosphorus deficiency is present. The deficiency almost always can be readily corrected by oral preparations containing phosphorus, and sometimes skim milk, a rich source of phosphorus, can be used as a dietary supplement.

The "psychiatric" symptoms of acute intermittent porphyria

The porphyrins are complex compounds that occur in all cells and are involved in storing and utilizing energy. The porphyrias are a group of disorders, usually hereditary, in which the body's handling of the porphyrins is disturbed. Some porphyrias are rare.

By far the most common is acute intermittent porphyria (AIP). It results from overproduction of porphyrin precursors—the materials that go into the making of porphyrins—in the liver.

AIP can manifest itself in childhood but most frequently

begins to do so between the ages of 20 and 40. And it does so in acute episodes with periods of freedom from all symptoms that sometimes are long.

Commonly in an attack there are colicky, often severe, abdominal pain, vomiting, distention, and diarrhea or constipation. Muscle pain is frequent. Sometimes, in some patients, convulsive seizures may occur.

Most patients develop mental and emotional disturbances varying from relatively mild, such as irritability and confusion, to severe, such as delirium and psychoses.

The disorder affects men less often than women. And the attacks sometimes can be related in women to the menstrual cycle and in both men and women may be triggered by weight-reducing diets, alcohol consumption, infections, and the use of any of a considerable number of drugs such as barbiturates, sulfa compounds, griseofulvin (an agent used for fungal infections), estrogen, other steroid hormones, and chlordiazepoxide (which is the one constituent of Librium, a tranquilizer used for tension and anxiety, and one of the ingredients in Librax, which is used for peptic ulcer and the irritable bowel syndrome).

AIP can be and has been confused with many things. Because of the abdominal colic, patients may have laparotomy (exploratory abdominal surgery) without diagnosis. AIP also has been mistaken for hysteria and psychiatric disturbance.

Yet, as authorities note, the presence of mental and emotional disturbances along with the abdominal symptoms should raise the suspicion of AIP. And there are various tests, including a blood test, which aid in diagnosis.

Various agents may be used. Chlorpromazine often can relieve abdominal symptoms during a very severe attack and helps relieve psychiatric symptoms. Reserpine is often helpful.

Diet alone—one high in carbohydrates—has been found to be often effective in minimizing attacks. And all the more so when barbiturates, fasting, alcohol, and other precipitating agents are avoided.

A physical basis for some delusional thinking

Paranoid delusions have long been thought to be the result of underlying thinking disorder—an inability to make reasonable inferences from data. It has been assumed that although evidence normally sufficient to destroy an unwarranted belief is available, the paranoid person persists in his belief in spite of it.

Among the explanations offered for delusional phenomena, the best known has been in terms of underlying sexual conflict advanced by Freud. In one way or another, such conflict presumably can disrupt the process of logical reasoning.

Another explanation, however, has been offered recently by Brendan A. Maher, chairman of Harvard University's Department of Psychology and Social Relations. Maher believes that the processes of inference are intact but impairment of function of a sensory input channel—hearing, for example—has distorted the evidence available to the patient.

In Maher's view, delusional beliefs are held not in the face of contrary evidence but because of evidence powerful enough to support them. The paranoid patient doesn't necessarily differ from a normal person in drawing inferences from evidence but in the kinds of perception from which inferences are to be drawn. And a normal observer, with no way to examine the patient's experience directly, often assumes that it is the same experience as his own and has to conclude that the patient's strange inferences are the results of faulty thinking.

As an example of the delusional process, Maher offers the case of the elderly person who becomes hard of hearing. As he has reported in the *Journal of Individual Psychology*, "The person experiences a gradual diminution in the loudness with which other people are speaking, and this readily lends itself to an interpretation that they are whispering.

Given this interpretation, the next problem for the subject is to understand why they are whispering and why they deny it when taxed with it.

"It is perfectly natural—given the interpretation of whispering—to conclude that an attempt is being made to conceal something from the listener. Thus a delusion of conspiracy is not only possible but eminently reasonable. Once this inference has been made, the chief remaining question is to understand what the object of the conspiracy is. If the individual has been authoritarian and punitive with his family, he may decide that they are planning revenge; if he is ashamed of some past or present activity of his own, he may conclude that it has been discovered; if he has exercised close control over the finances of the family, he may fear that there is a plot to deprive him of his money, and so on.

"What is of central importance to this rather simple situation is that the past history of the patient has not produced the delusion, the impairment of hearing has produced the delusion. Past history has merely helped to determine what the content of the delusion will be. The cure of the delusion is a hearing aid or a proper preliminary diagnosis of deafness. Psychotherapy directed at the content of the delusion may affect the patient's view of his own life history, but cannot eliminate the perception that other people are whispering, unless it is coupled with a recognition on the part of the patient that the trouble is an error of perception and does not lie in the external environment."

Support for Maher's theory of how paranoid delusions sometimes can develop comes from recent studies by two British physicians, A. F. Cooper and A. R. Curry, reported in the *Journal of Psychosomatic Research.*

In one study, Cooper and Curry looked into the rate of deafness among patients suffering from paranoia and others with an illness such as depression. The minimum criterion for deafness in the study was that the patient have difficulty in hearing speech in a group conversation or in an auditorium. The two investigators found that significantly more paranoid patients were deaf than were those with depression, and interviews with family members determined that among the paranoid the deafness had preceded the paranoia. The rate of deafness among the other patients did not differ from that in the general population.

In another study with the help of an ophthalmologist, the two investigators found that the rate of visual defects among paranoiacs is greater than in those with depression or other illness, suggesting that Maher's theory is not limited to explaining the delusions of the hard-of-hearing elderly.

Selected References

Chapter 1

Hall, R. C. W., et al.: "Psychiatric Symptoms Mask Physical Disorders." *Clinical Psychiatry News*, 5(8):43.

Behavioral Neurology Unit: *The Harvard Medical Area Focus*, 1/4/77.

Geschwind, N.: Reported in The Brain Prober. *Newsweek*, 12/20/76, p. 54.

Chapter 2

Yahraes, H.: *Psychological Factors in Organic Disease*. Publication of National Institute of Mental Health.

Galton, L.: *How Long Will I Live?* Macmillan, 1976.

Alexander, F., et al.: *Psychosomatic Specificity*. University of Chicago Press, 1968.

Schmale, A. H., Jr. *Psychosomatic Medicine*, 22:4, 1958.

Schmale, A. H., Jr., and Iker, H. P. *Psychosomatic Medicine*, 28:5, 1966.

Miller, B. F., and Galton, L.: *Freedom from Heart Attacks*. Simon and Schuster, 1972.

Selye, H.: *The Stress of Life*. McGraw-Hill, 1956.

Marcus, M. G.: "The Shaky Link Between Cancer and Character." *Psychology Today*, June 1976, p. 52.

Comroe, B. I.: "Follow-Up Study of 100 Diagnosed as Neurotic." *Journal of Nervous and Mental Disease*, 83:679, 1936.

Marshall, H.: "Incidence of Physical Disorders Among Psychiatric Inpatients." *British Medical Journal*, 2:468, 1949.
Meyer, B. C.: "Some Psychiatric Aspects of Surgical Practice." *Psychosomatic Medicine*, 20:203, 1958.
Herridge, C. F.: "Physical Disorders in Psychiatric Illness—A Study of 209 Consecutive Admissions." *Lancet*, ii:949, 1960.
Davies, D. W.: "Physical Illness in Psychiatric Out-Patients." *British Journal of Psychiatry*, 111:27, 1965.
Johnson, D. A. W.: "The Evaluation of Routine Physical Examinations in Psychiatric Cases." *Practitioner*, 200:686, 1968.
Maguire, G. P., and Granville-Grossman, K. L.: "Physical Illness in Psychiatric Patients." *British Journal of Psychiatry*, 115:1365, 1968.
Hall, R. C. W., et al.: "Physical Illness Presenting as Psychiatric Disease." American Psychosomatic Society, Atlanta, 1977.
Huapaya, L. V. M.: "Psychogenesis and Somatogenesis of Common Symptoms." *Canadian Medical Association Journal*, 112:1109, 1975.
Mai, F.: "Management of 'Psychosomatic' Problems in Clinical Practice." *Canadian Medical Association Journal*, 114; 684, 1976.
Saravay, S. M., and Koran, L. M.: "Organic Disease Mistakenly Diagnosed as Psychiatric." *Psychosomatics*, 18:6, 1977.

Chapter 3

Kline, N.: *From Sad to Glad.* Putnam, 1974.
Williams, J. G.: "Common Errors in the Treatment of Depression." *American Family Physician*, 14(2):60, 1976.
Hall, R. C. W., and Popkin, M. K.: "Psychological Symptoms of Physical Origin." *The Female Patient*, October 1977.
Rose, D. P.: "The Pill and Nutrition: A Most Intricate Relationship." *The Professional Nutritionist*, Summer 1977.
Strain, J. J., and Grossman, S. (eds.): *Psychological Care of the Mentally Ill.* Appleton-Century-Crofts, 1975.
Sachar, E. J.: "Evaluating Depression in the Medical Patient." In Strain and Grossman, *op. cit.*
Foster, F. G., et al.: "Rapid Eye Movement Sleep Density." *Archives of General Psychiatry*, 33:1119, 1976.
Coble, P., et al.: "Electroencephalographic Sleep Diagnosis of Primary Depression." *Archives of General Psychiatry*, 33:1124, 1976.
Kupfer, D. J.: "REM Latency: A Psychobiologic Marker for Primary Depressive Disease." *Biological Psychiatry*, 11:159, 1976.

Chapter 4

Hall, R. C. W., et al.: "Physical Illness Presenting as Psychiatric Disease." American Psychosomatic Society, Atlanta, 1977.
Martin, M.: "How Can the Physician Explain Anxiety." *Journal of the American Medical Association*, 238:1408, 1977.
Thompson, W. G.: "Drugs and Faith Healing." *Canadian Medical Association Journal*, 111:302, 1974.
Kiely, W. F.: "Psychiatric Syndromes in Critically Ill Patients." *Journal of the American Medical Association*, 235:2759, 1976.
Williams, J. G.: "Systematic Management of the Anxious Patient." *American Family Physician*, 15(2):124, 1977.
French, A. P., and Tupen, J. P.: "On a Relaxation Technique for Anxiety." *Journal of the American Medical Association*, 223:801, 1973.

Chapter 5

Botez, M. I., et al.: "Neurologic Disorders Responsive to Folic Acid Therapy." *Canadian Medical Association Journal*, 115:217, 1976.
Keen, S.: "Chasing the Blahs Away: Boredom and How to Beat It." *Psychology Today*, May 1977.
Galton, L.: *How Long Will I Live?* Macmillan, 1976.
Barnes, B. O.: *Hypothyroidism: The Unsuspected Illness.* Crowell, 1976.
Cheraskin, E., Ringsdorf, W. M., Jr., and Brecher, A.: *Psychodietetics.* Stein and Day, 1974.

Chapter 6

Greden, J. F.: "Anxiety or Caffeinism: A Diagnostic Dilemma." *American Journal of Psychiatry*, 131:1089, 1974.
———, et al.: "Mixed Anxiety and Depression Associated with Caffeinism Among Psychiatric Inpatients." Presented at the American Psychiatric Association annual meeting, 1977.
Editorial: "Anxiety Symptoms and Coffee Drinking." *British Medical Journal*, 1:296, 1975.
Winstead, D. K.: "Coffee Consumption Among Psychiatric Inpatients." *American Journal of Psychiatry*, 133:1447, 1976.

Chapter 7

Reports on Research, 2:1. On the urgency of anemia correction. Massachusetts Institute of Technology, Cambridge.

Titmuss, R. M.: *The Gift Relationship.* Pantheon, 1970.

Filer, L. E., Jr.: "The USA Today—Is It Free of Public Health Nutrition Problems? Anemia." *American Journal of Public Health,* 59:327.

Bryan, J. A., II: "Use and Abuse of Hematinics." *American Family Physician,* 7(6):121, 1973.

Galton, L.: *The Disguised Disease: Anemia.* Crown, 1975.

Silber, R.: Introduction to *The Disguised Disease: Anemia.* Crown, 1975.

Chapter 8

Jackson, A. E.: "Hypothyroidism." *Journal of the American Medical Association,* 165:121, 1957.

Kimball, O. P.: Hypothyroidism." *Kentucky Medical Journal,* 31:488, 1939.

Wharton, G. K.: "Unrecognized Hypothyroidism." *Canadian Medical Association Journal,* 40:371, 1939.

Ashner, R.: "Myxedematous Madness." *British Medical Journal,* 2:555, 1949.

Prange, A. J., et al.: "Enhancement of Imipramine Activity by Thyroid Hormone." *American Journal of Psychiatry,* 126:457, 1969.

Sanders, V.: "Neurologic Manifestations of Myxedema." *New England Journal of Medicine,* 226:599, 1962.

Whybrow, P. C., et al.: "Mental Changes Accompanying Thyroid Gland Dysfunction." *Archives of General Psychiatry,* 20:48, 1969.

Barnes, B. O.: *Hypothyroidism: The Unsuspected Illness.* Crowell, 1976.

Feldman, J. M.: "The Practical Use of Thyroid Tests." *American Family Physician,* 16(3):159, 1977.

Mills, L. C.: "Treatment of Hypothyroidism." *American Family Physician,* 14(5):170, 1976.

Krieger, D. T.: "Cushing's Syndrome: Diagnosis and Management." *Guidelines to Metabolic Therapy,* 6(2):1, 1977.

Merck Manual, 13th ed. 1977.

Chapter 9

Cohen, S.: "Sleep and Insomnia." *Journal of the American Medical Association,* 236:875, 1976.

Ayres, S., Jr.: "On the Serendipitous Discovery That Vitamin E Prevents Night Leg Cramps." *Executive Health,* 11:8, 1975. *Journal of Applied Nutrition,* 25:8, 1973. *Southern Medical Journal,* 67:1308, 1974.

Kennedy, H. P.: "Sleep Problems Dx Requires Day-Night Rhythm Check." *Medical Tribune,* 18(31):16, 1977.

Budzynski, T.: "Tuning in on the Twilight Zone." *Psychology Today,* August 1977.

Dement, W. C., Guilleminault, C., Hartmann, E., and Weitzman, E. D.: "Sleep and Sleep Disorders: A New Clinical Discipline." Albert Einstein College of Medicine Symposium, 1976.

Chapter 10

Greenberg, J.: "How Accurate Is Psychiatry?" *Science News,* 112:28, 1977.

Huapaya, L.: "Physical Symptoms of Psychological Origin and Psychological Symptoms of Organic or Physiological Origin." *St. Mary's Hospital Medical Bulletin,* 16:291, 1974.

Babb, R., and Eckman, P.: "Abdominal Epilepsy." *Journal of the American Medical Association,* 222:65, 1972.

Stevens, J. R.: "Psychiatric Implications of Psychomotor Epilepsy." *Archives of General Psychiatry,* 14:461, 1966.

Slater, E., and Beard, A. W.: "The Schizophrenia-like Psychosis of Epilepsy." *British Journal of Psychiatry,* 109:95, 1963.

Wells, C.: "Petit Mal Status Presenting as a Psychosis." *Transactions of the American Neurological Association,* 98:321, 1973.

LaWall, J.: "Psychiatric Presentations of Seizure Disorders." *American Journal of Psychiatry,* 133:3, 1976.

Adebimpe, V. R.: "Complex Partial Seizures Simulating Schizophrenia." *Journal of the American Medical Association,* 237:1339, 1977.

Chapter 11

Campbell, M. B.: "Neurologic Manifestations of Allergic Disease." *Annals of Allergy,* 31:485, 1973.

———: "Neurologic and Psychiatric Aspects of Allergy." *Otolaryngologic Clinics of North America*, 7:805, 1974.
Philpott, W. H., et al.: "The Four-Day Rotation of Foods." In *Clinical Ecology*, Dickey, L. D. (ed.). Thomas, 1976.
Randolph, T. J.: "Ecological Orientation Medicine." *Annals of Allergy*, 23:7, 1965.
Davison, H. M.: "Allergy of the Nervous System." *Quarterly Review of Allergy*, 6:157, 1952.
Rinkel, J. H., et al.: "The Diagnosis of Food Allergy." *Archives of Otolaryngology*, 79:87, 1964.
Mandell, M., and Rose, G. J.: "May Emotional Reactions Be Precipitated by Allergens?" *Connecticut Medicine*, 32:300, 1968.
Mandell, M.: "Cerebral Reactions in Allergic Patients." *Journal of International Academy of Metabiology*, 3:94, 1974.
Hughes, E., et al.: "Synthetic Nutrients Improve Allergy Testing." *Modern Medicine*, 45(5):33, 1977.

Chapter 12

Reed, B., and Shah, S.: As reported in "Can Chocolate Turn You Into a Criminal?" *The Wall Street Journal*, 6/2/77.
Levine, R.: "Hypoglycemia." *Journal of the American Medical Association*, 230:462, 1974.
Meloni, C. R.: "Hypoglycemia: What Kind of Problem Is It?" *American Family Physician*, 12(4):108, 1975.
Chandler, P. T.: "An Update on Reactive Hypoglycemia." *American Family Physician*, 16(5):113, 1977.
Brown, G. M.: "Psychiatric and Neurologic Aspects of Endocrine Disease." *Hospital Practice*, 10(8):71, 1975.
Saperstein, M. D., et al.: "The Hypoglycemic Dilemma." Panel discussion, American College of Physicians, Dallas, 1977.
Yudkin, J.: *Pure, White and Deadly*. Davis-Poynter, 1972.
Cheraskin, E., Ringsdorf, W. M., Jr., and Brecher, A.: *Psychodietetics*. Stein and Day, 1974.

Chapter 13

Snyder, J.: "National Commission Turns the Spotlight on Digestive Diseases." *Modern Medicine*, 45(15):17, 1977.
Thompson, W. G.: "The Irritable Colon." *Canadian Medical Association Journal*, 111:1236, 1974.
Texter, E. C., and Butler, R. C.: "The Irritable Bowel Syndrome." *American Family Physician*, 11(3):169, 1975.

Prout, B. S.: "The Irritable Colon Syndrome—Very Common But Often Missed." *Modern Medicine*, 45(13):36, 1977.
Manning, A. P., et al.: "Wheat Fibre and Irritable Bowel Syndrome: A Controlled Trial." *Lancet*, ii:417 (1977).
Galton, L.: *Save Your Stomach.* Crown, 1977.
———: *The Truth About Fiber in Your Food.* Crown, 1976.
Bayless, M.: "Recognition of Lactose Intolerance." *Hospital Practice*, 11(10):97, 1976.
Paige, D. M., et al.: "Lactose Hydrolyzed Milk." *American Journal of Clinical Nutrition*, 28:818, 1975.
Clearfield, H. R.: "Heartburn." *American Family Physician*, 15(2):158, 1977.
Stanciu, C., and Bennett, J. R.: "On Smoking and Heartburn." *British Medical Journal*, 3:793, 1972.

Chapter 14

Morgan, D. H.: "The Great Impostor: Diseases of the Temporomandibular Joint." *Journal of the American Medical Association*, 235:2395, 1976.
Shore, N. A.: "In Diagnosis of a Jaw Click." *Medical Tribune*, 18(24):9, 1977.
———: *Temporomandibular Joint Dysfunction and Occlusal Equilibration*, 2nd ed. Lippincott, 1976.
Gelb, H., and Tarte, J.: "A Two-Year Dental Evaluation of 200 Cases of Chronic Headache." *Journal of the American Dental Association*, 91:1230, 1975.
Dohrmann, R. J.: "Treatment of Myofascial Pain Dysfunction Syndrome with EMG Feedback." International Association for Dental Research, 1976.
Kudrow, L.: "On Migraine and Estrogen." *Headache*, 15:36, 1976.
Dalessio, D. J.: "On Migraine and Diet." *American Family Physician*, 6(6):60, 1972.
Gilbert, G. J.: "On 'Turtle' Headaches." *Journal of the American Medical Association*, 221:1165, 1972.

Chapter 15

Reichel, W.: "Multiple Problems in the Elderly." *Hospital Practice*, 11(3):103, 1976.
———: "Organic Brain Syndrome in the Aged." *Hospital Practice*, 11(5):119, 1976.
Arehart-Treichel, J.: "Senility: More Than Growing Old." *Science News*, 112:29, 1977.

Henig, R. M.: "Tomorrow's Challenge: Health Care for the Elderly." *The New Physician*, 26(10):25, 1977.
Brink, T. L.: "The Battle Against Senility." *Mental Hygiene*, 61(2):11, 1977.
Walsh, A. C. and B. H.: "Presenile Dementia: Further Experience with an Anticoagulant-Psychotherapy Regimen." *Journal of the American Geriatrics Society*, 22:467, 1974.
"Psychosomatic Treatment Counteracts Senility." *Science News*, 111:292, 1977.
Haynes, C. D.: "Surgery Helps Mental Status of Some Patients." Medical News Section, *Journal of the American Medical Association*, 236:2037, 1976.
Ferguson, G. G.: "Cerebrovascular Dementia Reversible by Anastomosis." *Medical Tribune*, 17(18):43, 1976.
Charlton, M. H.: "Presenile Dementia." *New York State Journal of Medicine*, 75:1493, 1975.

Chapter 16

Sterner, R. T., and Price, W. R.: "Restricted Riboflavin Within-Subject Behavioral Effects in Humans." *American Journal of Clinical Nutrition*, 26:150, 1973.
Dans, W. H., and Zlady, F.: "Symptoms Related to Mineral Deficiencies." 2nd International Symposium on Magnesium, Montreal, 1976.
Whang, R., et al.: "Routine Serum Magnesium Determination—An Unrecognized Need." Montreal Symposium.
Brin, M.: "Marginal Deficiency States of Water Soluble Vitamins." Symposium on Micronutrients, New Orleans, 1977.
Truswell, A. S., et al.: "Thiamine Deficiency in Adult Hospital Patients." *South African Medical Journal*, 46:2079, 1972.
Hawkins, D., and Pauling, L.: *Orthomolecular Psychiatry*. Freeman, 1973.
Roe, D. A.: *Drug-Induced Nutritional Deficiencies*. Avi Publishing Co., 1976.
Food and Nutrition Board. "Proposed Fortification Policy for Cereal Grain Products." National Academy of Science/National Research Council, Washington, D.C., 1974.
"Nutrition—No Longer a Stepchild in Medicine." Medical News Section, *Journal of the American Medical Association*, 238:2245, 1977.

Chapter 17

Walker, A. R. P.: "Too Many Pills." *Canadian Medical Association Journal,* 115:382, 1976.
Detzer, E., et al.: "Identifying and Treating the Drug-Misusing Patient." *American Family Physician,* 16(3):181, 1977.
Galton, L.: *The Complete Book of Symptoms.* Simon and Schuster, 1978.

Chapter 18

Mathew, N. T.: "On Blood Fat Levels and Neuropathies." Report to American Academy of Neurology, 1976.
Smith, J. R., and Landaw, S. A.: "Smokers' Polycythemia." *New England Journal of Medicine,* 298:6, 1978.
"Rx for Familial Mediterranean Fever." *Medical World News,* 15(26):35, 1974.
"On Systemic Lupus Erythematosus." Report from National Jewish Hospital and Research Center, Denver, 1977.
"On Wilson's Disease": *Merck Manual,* 13th ed. 1977.
Lum, L. C.: "Hyperventilation: The Tip and the Iceberg." *Journal of Psychosomatic Research,* 19:375, 1975.
Shapiro, A. K. and E.: "Gilles de la Tourette's Syndrome." *American Family Physician,* 9(6):94, 1974.
Golden, G. S.: "Tourette Syndrome." *American Journal of Diseases of Children,* 131:531, 1977.
Kreisberg, R. A.: "Phosphorus Deficiency and Hypophosphatemia." *Hospital Practice,* 12(3):121, 1977.
Maher, B.: "Delusional Thinking and Perceptual Disorder." *Journal of Individual Psychology,* 30:98, 1977.
Cooper, A. F., and Curry, A. R.: "On Paranoia and Deafness." *Journal of Psychosomatic Research,* 20:97, 1976.
Cooper, A. F., and Porter, R.: "On Paranoia and Visual Defects." *Journal of Psychosomatic Research,* 20:107, 1976.

Index

About the Author

LAWRENCE GALTON is a noted medical writer and editor and a former visiting professor at Purdue University. He is a columnist for the Washington Star Syndicate and *Family Circle,* and his articles frequently appear in *The New York Times Magazine, Reader's Digest, Parade,* and other national publications. He is the author of more than a dozen other books.